NAME SUB TITTLE

The Complete Bariatric Cookbook and Meal Plan

+100 Simple and Tasty Recipes for Lifelong Health

Sajibahmed

TABLE OF CONTENTS

The Full Guide to Gastric Bypass Surgery

Contents Table of Contents

Gastric bypass surgery will save your life. You will slim down. Your co-morbidities would be diminished. You'll feel and look healthier as a result. However, in order to be successful (in the long run), you must change your diet.

This seems to be a straightforward mission, but it is not. Prepare yourself for a war. You've spent a large part of your life promoting and reinforcing unhealthy eating habits. Those must be changed.

The first step toward a balanced diet is to realize what you can and cannot consume. For two reasons, the diet for the first five weeks after gastric bypass surgery is critical.

Your wellbeing is paramount. Eating the wrong foods will put excessive strain on your stomach as it heals.

Getting rid of unhealthy eating habits and replacing them with new, better ones.

Liquid Diet Prior to Surgery

A preoperative liquid diet must be practiced 7-14 days before gastric bypass surgery to reduce the volume of fat around the liver and spleen. If this diet is not practiced, surgery will be deferred or cancelled during the operation (during the procedure).

The value of adhering to the pre-op diet cannot be overstated. You've typically waited anywhere from 6 to 12 months to be accepted and on the operating table. Keep to a pre-op diet.

Water and a diet log

A large liver makes it impossible for the surgeon to see such anatomy during the operation. It is risky to perform gastric bypass surgery if the liver is too large. Surgery could be postponed and rescheduled for a later time.

The following items will be used in the 1-2 week pre-op diet:

The diet's mainstay will be protein shakes or meal substitute shakes.

Only non-sugar drinks are approved (sugar substitutes are okay).

There are no caffeinated or carbonated drinks allowed.

It is acceptable to eat soup broth that contains no solid bits of food.

Vegetable juice and V8 are also suitable choices.

Cream of wheat or rice that is very thin can also be consumed.

One or two daily servings of lean meat and/or vegetables can be permissible, but only if your physician or licensed dietician agrees.

Both drinks and beverages should be sipped steadily. Beverages should not be eaten with meals, and the patient should wait at least 30 minutes after eating to drink something.

BARIATRIC RECIPE

1.THE FULL GUIDE TO GASTRIC BYPASS SURGERY

SERVES 2 .COOKS IN: 15 MINUTES

Ingredients

- vegetable oil
- 4 large free-range eggs
- SPINACH & HAM
- 20 g baby spinach
- 75 g quality cooked ham
- TOMATO & BASIL
- 70 g ripe cherry tomatoes
- 1 sprig of fresh basil
- SMOKED SALMON & CHIVES
- 50 g smoked salmon
- a few fresh chives
- TRUFFLE MUSHROOMS
- 50 g mushrooms chestnut
- truffle oila few drops of

Method

1. Preheat the boiler to full whack. Grease 2 ovenproof ramekins or shallow baking dishes lightly with a small amount of oil.

2. Prepare your desired filling – loosely chop the lettuce, quarter the tomatoes, thinly chop the chives or dice the mushrooms.

3. Place your preferred filling into the prepared ramekins, crack a couple of eggs on top and season with salt and pepper.

4. Place in the hot oven for 8 to 10 minutes, or until the whites are set but the yolks are still runny, then serve straight awayPreheat the oven to full whack. Grease 2 ovenproof ramekins or shallow baking dishes lightly with a small amount of oil.

5. Prepare your desired filling – loosely chop the lettuce, quarter the tomatoes, thinly chop the chives or dice the mushrooms.

6. Place your preferred filling into the prepared ramekins, crack a couple of eggs on top and season with salt and pepper.

7. Place for 8 to 10 minutes in the hot oven

8. NUTRITION PER SERVING

Calories233

2.TURKEY BREAKFAST SAUSAGE\

Prep:10 mins

Cook:10 mins

Total:20 mins

Ingredients

- 2 pounds ground turkey
- 1 tbsp brown sugar
- 2 tsp kosher salt
- 1 ½ tsp ground black pepper
- 1 ½ tsp ground sage
- 1 ½ tsp ground thyme
- ½ tsp dried marjoram
- ½ tsp red pepper flakes

Directions

1. Mix turkey, brown sugar, cinnamon, black pepper, sage, thyme, marjoram, and red pepper flakes in a bowl. Shape a combination of turkey into patties.
2. Fry patties in a large skillet over medium-high heat until golden brown and no longer pink in the middle, 6 to 8 minutes.

Nutrition Facts:

176 calories.

3.GRILLED CHEESE DE MAYO

Prep:10 mins

Cook:33

5 mins

Total:15 mins

Ingredients

- 1 tbspdivided mayonnaise
- 2 slices white bread
- 2 slices American cheese
- 1 slice pepperjack cheese

Directions

1. On one side of a bread slice, spread 1/2 of the mayonnaise and place it in a skillet, mayonnaise-side down. With the pepperjack cheese, place the American cheese on top of the bread. Spread the rest of the mayonnaise into a single slice.

Nutrition Facts:

500 calories.

4.HASH BROWNS

Preparation time

30 mins to 1 hour

Cooking time

10 to 30 mins

Ingredients

- 4 medium peeled floury potatoes
- 1 medium onion
- 1 egg, beaten
- salt and pepper
- vegetable oil, for frying

Method

1.Coarsely grind the potatoes and onion into a clean tea towel and then squeeze out the remaining moisture by twisting the towel. Place the mix in a wide bowl.

2.Add the egg, a decent couple of pinches of salt and freshly ground black pepper (you need to salt the mixture well.

3.Heat a decent glug of oil in a heavily based frying pan and when the oil is hot (but not smoking), add spoonfuls of the potato mixture into the pan and flatten into patties around 1cm/½in deep. Flip over until browned and crispy – around 2–3 minutes per hand.

4.Serve hot as a breakfast .

5.MAMA KAYE'S SALMON BREAKFAST CROQUETTES

Total: 1 hr 35 min

Prep: 15 min

Inactive: 1 hr

Cook: 20 min

Ingredients

- Deselect All
- 8 ounces baked or poached salmon, flaked
- 2 largebeaten eggs
- 2 cups of mashed potatoes
- 1 smalldiced white onion
- 5 minced cloves garlic
- Salt and pepper
- 6 tbsp all-purpose flour
- Peanut oil, for frying

Directions

1. In a large bowl, combine the salmon, eggs, mashed potatoes, onion and garlicSeason with salt and pepper. To hold the paste together, whisk in the rice.

2. Form into golf-ball-size spheres with the combination. Refrigerate overnight or for 1 hour.

3. In a big straight-sided skillet, heat around 1 inch of peanut oil until a deep-fry thermometer registers 325 degrees. Fry the croquettes, in batches, for 3 to 4 minutes, until crisp and golden on one side, adjusting as desired. On the other side, turn and cook until golden, for 1 to 2 more minutes. Drain yourself on paper towels

My Private Notes

6.CHEESY BREAKFAST EGG ROLLS

Total Time

Prep: 30 min. Cook: 10

Ingredients

- 1/2 pound bulk pork sausage
- 1/2 cup of shredded sharp cheddar cheese
- 1/2 cup of shredded Monterey Jack cheese
- 1 tbsp chopped green onions
- 4 large eggs
- 1 tbsp 2% milk
- 1/4 tsp salt
- 1/8 tsp pepper
- 1 tbsp butter
- 12 egg roll wrappers
- Cooking spray
- Maple syrup

Directions

1. In a small nonstick skillet, cook sausage over medium heat until no longer pink, 4-6 minutes, breaking into crumbles; rinse. Stir in cheeses and green onions; set aside. Wipe skillet clean.

2. In a shallow bowl, mix eggs, milk, salt and pepper until mixed Melt the butter in the same pan over a low fire.. Pour in egg mixture; cook and stir until eggs are thickened and no liquid egg remains. Stir in sausage mixture.
3. Preheat air fryer to 400°. With 1 corner of an egg roll wrapper facing you, position 1/4 cup of filling just below center of wrapperFold the bottom corner over the filling and wet the remaining water wrapper edges. Fold side corners against middle over filling. Roll egg roll up firmly, pulling at tip to seal. Repeat.

4. Place the egg rolls in batches on the greased tray in the air-fryer basket in a single layer sprinkle with the cooking spray. For 3-4 minutes, cook until lightly browned. Turn; spritz with water for frying. Cook until golden brown and crisp, for 3-4 more minutes. Serve with maple syrup or salsa if desired.

Nutrition Facts:

209 calories.

7.EASY COCONUT SHRIMP

Prep Time: 20 minutes Cook Time: 10 minutes Total Time: 30 minutes

Ingredients

- 1/3 cup of all-purpose flour or whole wheat flour
- 1/2 tsp salt
- 1/2 tsp ground black pepper
- 2 largebeaten eggs
- 3/4 cup of Panko bread crumbs
- 1 cup of sweetened shredded coconut
- 1 pound raw large shrimp, peeled and deveined with tails attached
- vegetable oil

Instructions

1. Start off with three medium bowls. Mix in the rice, salt, and pepper.In the second bowl beat the eggsIn the third bowl, combine the Panko and the coconut.

2. Dip the shrimp into the rice, then the eggs, then dredge the shrimp into the mixture of the coconut, pressing softly to hold to it. On some shrimp, you like a lot of coconut. On a pan, set the coated shrimp aside while you coat the remaining shrimp.

3. To coat the bottom of a large skillet over medium heat, add enough oil. Do not crowd them in the pan by cooking the coconut shrimp in clusters. I fried 6-7 of them at a time. Flip after 2 minutes and cook for 2 minutes or until golden brown on the other hand. I like mine a little darker, so I've been frying either hand for about three minutes now.

4. On a plate lined with a paper towel, place the finished coconut shrimp while you fry the remainder. Serve with your own sweet chili sauce or orange chili sauce (1 part orange marmalade of Thai sweet chili sauce for 2 parts) (which is 1 part Thai sweet chili sauce to 2 parts orange marmalade). I tried this dipping sauce, and it is also very tasty.

5. Sprinkle and serve with a little chopped cilantro (optional).
For up to 3 days, the leftover coconut shrimp remains well in the refrigerator.

Notes

- ok, up to 2 months. Reheat for 10 minutes in a 350°F (177°C) oven– or until thawed and warm.
- Coconut Oil: I prefer frying the coconut shrimp in coconut oil for the best ta!

FISH& SEAFOOD

8.BAKED TUNA STEAK

PREP TIME:10 mins

COOK TIME:30 mins

TOTAL TIME:40 mins

INGREDIENTS

- 1 tsp salt
- ¼ tsp black pepper
- 2minced cloves garlic
- ¼ tsp red pepper flakes
- 4 small tuna steaks
- ½ cup of olive oil
- ¼ cup of lemon juice
- 2 tbsp teriyaki sauce

INSTRUCTIONS

1. Preheat the oven to 375°F

2. Combine well and rub together the salt, vinegar, garlic and pepper flakes on both sides of the tuna steak.

3. In a shallow baking dish, make two tablespoons of olive oil and lay on tuna steaks

4. Combine the remaining 6 tablespoons of olive oil, lemon juice and teriyaki sauce, and substitute the tuna. Bake with a fork for 30 minutes or before the fish flakes quickly. Baste with a mixture of seasoned oil 2 to 3 times during baking.

9.CUMIN-LIME SHRIMP WITH GINGER

YIELD4 servings

TIME15 minutes

INGREDIENTS

- 1 ½ poundspeeled and deveined shrimp,
- 1 tsp ground cumin
- Kosher salt
- 3 tbsp olive oil
- 1 ½ tsp grated ginger
- 1 tsp grated garlic
- Pinch of red-pepper flakes
- ¼ cup of lime juice
- 1 tsp lime zest
- 3 tbsp roughly chopped cilantro
- Flaky salt

PREPARATION

1.Toss together the shrimp and the cumin in a wide bowl until well seasoned. Using kosher salt to season and toss again.

2. Over medium heat, heat the olive oil in a 12-inch skillet. In one layer, add half the shrimp to the pan and cook undisturbed until it just begins to turn pink, around 1 minute. Flip for about 1 more minute and cook, then remove from the pan and set aside. At this time, they might not be fully cooked, and that's O.K. Repeat and leave in the pan with the remaining shrimp.

3. For any juices that have accumulated, add the preserved shrimp back to the skillet. Stir in the flakes of ginger, garlic and red pepper, if used, and boil for around 30 seconds, stirring till the garlic does not burn. At the bottom of the plate, add the lime juice to the pan and scrape away any brown bits that have gathered. Cook until about half of the mixture is reduced, about an additional 1 minute. Stir in the zest of the lime and sprinkle the cilantro with it. If required, season with flaky salt.

MEAT RECIPES

10.STEAK SALAD

Prep Time:35 mins

Cook Time:10 mins

Total Time:45 mins

Servings:4 servings

Ingredients

- Balsamic Vinaigrette
- ¼ cup of balsamic vinegar
- 2tspdijon mustard
- 1 tsp mayonnaise, optional
- ½ tsp kosher salt

- ¼ tsp black pepper
- ½ cup of extra-virgin olive oil
- Steak Salad
- 1 poundflank steak, or flat iron steak
- kosher salt, for seasoning
- black pepper, for seasoning
- 2 tbsp olive oil
- 4 cups of arugula, 1-inch pieces
- 4 cups of romaine lettuce
- 2 cups of radicchio, 1-inch pieces
- 1 cup of cherry tomatoes, cut in half
- ½ cup of thinly sliced cucumber
- ¼ cup of thinly sliced radish
- ¼ cup of diced red onion
- 1 medium sliced avocado
- ¼ cup of feta cheese

Instructions

1. In a medium bowl stir together vinegar, mustard, mayonnaise, salt, and pepper.
2. Slowly drizzle in the olive oil and whisk until it becomes a thickened emulsified dressing.
3. Dry the top of the steak with paper towels.
4. Season all sides with salt and pepper.
5. Heat a large cast-iron skillet over high heat until hot. Add the oil, once the oil is hot add the steak and press it back into the grill. Cook until the surface is browned, 4 minutes.
6. Flip the steak and cook until it reveryes an internal temperature of 120 to 125°F (49 to 52ºC) for medium-rare, around 3 to 5 minutes.

7. Transfer the steak to a cutting board and rest for 10 minutes. Slice the steak against the grain into ¼-inch thick sections. Split narrower if needed.

8. In a wide serving bowl blend together the arugula, romaine, and radicchio.

9. Top salad with tomatoes, cucumber, radish, cabbage, steak, avocado, and feta cheeseServe steak salad with balsamic vinaigrette.

Nutrition Facts

Calories from Fat 450

11.MINUTE STEAK WITH CHIPOTLE BUTTER AND LIME

TIME: 30 mins

SERVES:4 with leftover butter

- ### *Ingredients*
- 400g beef eye fillet, preferably centre cut
- sea salt and freshly ground black pepper
- olive oil
- 4 fresh lime cheeks
- For the butter
- 250g unsalted butter, very soft
- 1 chipotle chilli in chopped adobo sauce
- 1 tspsalt sea
- ¾ tsppaprika smoky
- 1 tsp freshlytoasted ground cumin
- freshly ground black pepper

Method

1. Bring all the ingredients to a mixing bowl for the butter and combine until smooth with a wooden spoon. Spoon on some cling film, then roll around 5cm in diameter into a log. Place until solid in the refrigerator, then cut into 1/2cm strips. Set aside 4 slices of ample sliced butter, placing each slice on a baking paper square. The butter must be at room temperature, so that the steak melts easily.

2. For later usage, send the remaining butter to the fridge or freezer. When frozen, between each slice, place a small piece of baking paper so that you can use it, slice by slice, when and when you need it.

3. Cut the beef into four steaks crosswise. Place some slice, one by one, between 2 sheets of film cling and pound, until very thin (about 5 mm) (about 5mm). Remove the cling film and season the beef with black pepper and sea salt, then lightly drizzle with the oil.

4. On a high heat, preheat a grill or frying pan. Cook on one side (until browned) for around 1 minute per slice of beef, then turn and cook for another 10 seconds - it should still be juicy and pink in the middle. Remove from heat, cover with foil, and take a minute to relax.

5. Cover the cooked minute steak with a slice of softened butter and immediately serve with fresh lime.

6. Tip: I prefer eating this dish with raw cabbage and cucumber salad and rolling it all up in a tortilla.

12.STEAK AND PEPPERS

Prep Time: 10 minutes

<u>Cook</u> Time: 1 hour

Total Time: 1 hour 10 minutes

Ingredients

- 2 pounds round steak
- 2 tblsp canola oil
- 2 cups of beef broth
- ¼ tspgarlic powder
- ½ tsp salt
- ½ tsp ground ginger
- 1 large green pepper
- 1 large onion
- 1 tblsp cornstarch
- 2 tblsp water
- 1 tblspsoy sauce

Instructions

1Remove and discard the fat that reaches. Cut the meat into strips of nearly 1 "x 3".

2. Over high pressure, heat the oil in a large deep frying pan.

3. Stir in the beef and grill until it is browned

4. Incorporate the beef broth, stirring well.

5. Garlic powder, salt, and ginger are applied and combine well.

6. Bring the flame to a boil, reduce it, and cover the pan. Bake for 30 minutes at a boil.

7. By cutting them both into thin slices, prepare the onion(s) and pepper.

8. For an additional 30 minutes or until the vegetables are tender and the meat is cooked through, add the onions and pepper to the pan, bring back to a boil, lower the heat and simmer.

9. In a small dish, mix the cornstarch, water and soy sauce together.

Oh. 10. Before the sauce is thickened, add it to the pan and boil for a few minutes.

11. Over hot steamed rice, eat.

Notes

- Nutrition knowledge is determined by algorithms based on the ingredients of a recipe. It is an approximation only and is given for explanatory purposes. You can contact your health care professional or a registered dietitian if detailed nutrition measurements are required for health purposes.

Nutrition

Calories: 680kcal

13.APRICOT BROWN SUGAR HAM

Cook:2 hrs

Total:2 hrs

Servings:15

Ingredients

- 10 pound fully-cooked spiral cut ham

- ⅔ cup of brown sugar
- ⅓ cup of apricot jam
- 1 tsp dry mustard powder

Directions

1. Preheat the furnace to 135 degrees C (275 degrees F) (135 degrees C).

2. Set the cut side of the ham down on a sheet of aluminum foil. I'd like to pull out the shiny side. In a small cup, blend the brown sugar, apricot jelly and mustard powder together. Using a pastry or barbeque brush to paste on to the ham. Reserve the glaze that remains. Enclose the foil and place on a rimmed baking sheet around the ham.

3. Roast in a preheated oven for 2 hours, or if the size of the ham is different, measure 14 minutes per pound. 20 minutes before the ham is full, apply the remaining glaze.

Nutrition Facts

801 calories

14.TERIYAKI PORK STIR FRY

Prep Time10 minutes

Cook Time20 minutes

Total Time30 minutes

INGREDIENTS

- 1 tbsp vegetable oil divided use
- 1 cup of broccoli florets
- 1/2 cupthinly sliced of carrots
- 3/4 cup of bell peppers cut into
- 1 inch pieces, I used red and yellow
- 1 pound pork tenderloin cut into
- 1 inchminced pieces 1 tsp ginger
- 2 tspminced garlic
- 1 tbsp sesame seeds
- salt and pepper as need
- For the sauce
- 1/4 cup of soy sauce
- 1/2 cup of water
- 3 tbsp brown sugar
- 1 tbsp honey
- 1 tsp toasted sesame oil
- 1 tbsp cornstarch

INSTRUCTIONS

1. Heat 1 teaspoon of oil over medium-high heat in a large pan. Add the broccoli, peppers and carrots and roast for 4-6 minutes until finely browned and softened. As required, season with salt and pepper.

2. Remove the vegetables from the pan; to remain warm, place on a plate and cover with foil.

3. Add the remaining 2 TSP of oil to the pan. Add the pork and, if needed, season with salt and pepper. Cook, stirring occasionally, for 4-6 minutes, until the meat is browned and cooked.

4. In the pan, add the garlic and ginger and boil for 30 seconds.

5. Render the sauce as the pork is pan fried. In a small pot over medium-high heat, place the soy sauce, water, brown sugar, honey and sesame oil. Stir for about 3 minutes before the sugar is dissolved. Turn the fire to an intense degree and get it to a boil.

6. Till it is dissolved, mix 2 tbsp of cold water with the cornstarch. Apply this paste of cornstarch to the sauce and steam for 1-2 minutes, or before the sauce thickens.

7. With the bacon, add the vegetables back to the skillet. Pour in the sauce and coat it with a toss. To scatter, use sesame seeds, then serve.

NUTRITION

Calories: 278kcal

15.CAJUN CHICKEN BREAST

Prep Time: 5 minutesCook Time: 10 minutes

Ingredients

- 2 lbs chicken breasts 3 large, boneless & skinless
- 1 tbsp avocado oil
- Homemade Cajun Seasoning:
- 2 1/2 tsp paprika
- 2 tsp garlic powder
- 1 1/4 tsp oregano
- 1 1/4 tsp thyme
- 1 tsp onion powder
- 1 tsp cayenne pepper
- 1 tsp ground black pepper
- 1 1/2 tsp salt
- 1/2 tsp red pepper flakes

Instructions

1.Cut the chicken breasts into thinner cutlets lengthwise and position them in a large bowl. Add paprika, garlic powder, oregano, thyme, onion powder, cayenne pepper, black pepper, salt and flakes of red pepper to a small bowl; mix to blend.

2. In the step above, spray 1 1/2 tbsp of seasoned cajun seasoning on chicken breasts and use tongs to cover them. You can also add avocado oil to the mix whether you are grilling or baking Cajun chicken.

3. Pan Fried Cajun Chicken: Preheat medium-heat large ceramic non-stick skillet and brush with swirl oil. Cook for 5 minutes or before white edges appear, turn and cook for another 4-5 minutes. Add chicken and cook.

4. Cajun Chicken Baked: Preheat the oven to 450 degrees F, place the chicken in a large baking dish in a single layer and bake for 25 minutes. Remove from the oven, cover and leave for about 10 minutes to relax.

5. Grilled Cajun Chicken: Preheat the grill to 450-500 degrees F (medium-high heat), place the chicken on the grill, close the lid and grill for 8-10 minutes, turning once. Do not overcook anymore. Remove from the grill, cover with foil, and leave for around 5 minutes to relax.

Notes

- Cajun spice mix is from Allrecipes.comCajun spice mix is from Allrecipes.com

NUTRITION

Calories: 201kcal

16.KOREAN FRIED CHICKEN

YIELDS:4 SERVINGS

PREP TIME:0 HOURS 15 MINS

TOTAL TIME:1 HOUR 0 MINS

INGREDIENTS

- Vegetable oil
- 1 tsp kosher salt
- 1/2 tsp freshly ground black pepper
- 1/2 tsp baking powder
- 1/2 tsppowder garlic
- 2 lb chicken wings
- 1 tbsp freshly grated ginger
- 1/2 ccornstarch

DIRECTIONS

1. Make the wings: In a deep pot over medium-high heat, heat 4 to 6 cups of vegetable oil to 275 °. Cover a large plate or baking sheet with paper towels. In a shallow bowl, mix the salt, pepper, baking powder, and garlic powder.

2. Dry the pat wings with paper towels, then brush with grated ginger and season with the salt mixture. In a wide bowl, throw cornstarch wings and pinch to compress the coating onto either wing.

3. Carefully add the wings to the oil and cook until the skin is finely crisped and golden, frequently tossed with tongs, for around 15 to 18 minutes. Set the prepared tray aside and remove the wings from the oil. Let's pause momentarily.

4. Gas the cooking oil at 400°. Place the wings back in the pot and fried again for about 7 to 8 minutes, until the skin is crisp and crunchy and intensely golden,Take out the oil with the wings and place them in a large mixing bowl.

5. Make the sauce: In a medium saucepan over medium-low heat, mix the butter, dried chilis, ginger and garlic and cook until fragrant, for 2 minutes. Before bubbling, stir in gochujang, ketchup, soy sauce, and vinegar and simmer. Stir in honey and brown sugar and finish boiling until somewhat thickened and bubbling.

6. Over the sauce, pour the wings and toss until the wings are finely colored. To mix, add the peanuts and stir.

7. Garnish it with sesame and green onion seeds before feeding.

17.CHICKEN TIKKA MASALA

PREP:15 MINS

COOK:30 MINS

TOTAL:45

INGREDIENTS

- For the chicken marinade:
- 28 oz boneless and skinless chicken thighs cut into bite-sized pieces
- 1 cup of plain yogurt
- 1 1/2 tbsp minced garlic
- 1 tbsp ginger
- 2 tsp garam masala
- 1 tsp turmeric
- 1 tsp ground cumin

- 1/2 tsp ground red chili powder
- 1 tsp of salt
- For the sauce:
- 2 tbsp of vegetable/canola oil
- 2 tbsp butter
- 2 smallfinely diced onions
- 1 1/2 tbspfinely grated garlic
- 1 tbspfinely grated ginger
- 1 1/2 tsp garam masala
- 1 1/2 tsp ground cumin
- 1 tsp turmeric powder
- 1 tsp ground coriander
- 14 oz tomato puree
- 1 tsp Kashmiri chili
- 1 tsp ground red chili powder
- 1 tsp salt
- 1 1/4 cups of heavy
- 1 tsp brown sugar
- 1/4 cup of water if needed
- 4 tbsp Fresh cilantro or coriander to garnish

INSTRUCTIONS

1. Mix chicken with all the chicken marinade ingredients in a bowl; leave to marinate for 10 minutes to an hour (or overnight if time permits) (or overnight if time permits) (or overnight if time allows).

2. Heat oil over medium-high heat in a large skillet or a kettle. Add chicken pieces in batches of two or three when sizzling, making sure not to crowd the grill. Fry until browned for just 3 minutes on either side. Throw yourself aside and stay warm. (In the sauce, you should finish cooking the chicken.)

3. Melt the butter in the same panFry the onions until smooth (about 3 minutes) while wiping up any browned bits stuck on the bottom of the pan.

4. Add the garlic and ginger and sauté until fragrant for 1 minute, then mix in the garam masala, cumin, turmeric and cilantro. Fry until fragrant for about 20 seconds, while stirring occasionally.

5. Pour in the tomato puree, salt and chili powder. Let it boil for about 10-15 minutes, stirring occasionally before thickening the sauce and turning a dark red brown colour.

6. Stir the milk and sugar through the sauce. Back in the pan, add the chicken and its juices and cook for a further 8-10 minutes before the chicken is cooked and the sauce is thick and bubbling. If needed, pour in the water to thin out the sauce.

7. Garnish with cilantro and serve with hot buttered garlic rice and fresh homemade Naan bread.

NUTRITION

Calories: 580kcal

18.MAPLE ROAST TURKEY PREP:

Cook:3 hrs 30 mins

Additional:2 hrs

Total:6 hrs 30 mins

Servings:12

Ingredients

- 2 cups of apple cider
- ⅓ cup of real maple syrup
- 2 ½ tbsp chopped fresh thyme
- 2 tbsp chopped fresh marjoram
- 1 ½ tsp grated lemon zest
- ¾ cup of butter, softened
- salt and pepper as need
- 12 pound whole turkey, neck and giblets reserved
- 2 cups of chopped onion
- 1 ½ cups of chopped celery
- 1 ½ cups of chopped carrots
- 3 cups of chickenbroth
- ¼ cup of all-purpose flour
- 1 bay leaf
- ½ cup of apple brandy

Directions

1. In a saucepan, combine the apple cider and maple syrup and bring it to a boil over medium-high heat. Continue to cook until it is reduced to 1/2 cup, then remove the heat from the pan. Incorporate 1 tablespoon of thyme, 1 tablespoon of marjoram, and lemon zest. Stir in the butter and season with salt and pepper until it is melted. Cover and, until cool, refrigerate.

2. Preheat oven to 375 degrees F (190 degrees C) (190 degrees C) (190 degrees C) Add the rack to the lower third of the oven.

3. Place the turkey in a roasting pan on a stand. Reserve 1/4 cup of maple butter for gravy, and rub the remaining maple butter under the skin of the breast and over the outside of turkey. Arrange the turkey around the cabbage, celery, onions, turkey neck and giblets. Sprinkle over the vegetables with 1 tbsp of thyme and 1 tbsp of marjoram. Pour the pan into 2 cups of broth.

4. Roast turkey for 30 minutes in the preheated ovenReduce the temperature of the oven to 175 degrees C (350 degrees F) (175 degrees C). Lightly coat the whole turkey with foil. Continue roasting for about 2 1/2 hours or until the meat thermometer has 180 degrees F (85 degrees C) inserted into the thickest portion of the leg (85 degrees C). Transfer the turkey to the pan and leave stand for 30 minutes.

5.Strain the juices into a large large beaker from the pan and drain any excess fat. To weigh 3 cups, add enough chicken broth to the pan juices. Place the liquid in a saucepan and bring it to a boil. Mix 1/4 cup maple butter and 1/3 cup flour in a small bowl until smooth. Whisk the combination of flour and butter into the broth. Stir in the remaining bay leaf and the thyme. Boil until the consistency of the sauce is reduced, stirring occasionally, for about 10 minutes. If needed, blend in the apple brandy. Use salt and pepper to season as needed.

1. ***Nutrition Facts***

872 calories

19.CHICKEN PICCATA

otal: 40 min

Prep: 15 min

Cook: 25 min

Yield: 4 servings

Ingredients

- Deselect All
- 2 skinless and boneless chicken breasts, butterflied and then cut in half
- Sea salt and freshlyblack pepper ground
- All-purpose flour for dredging
- 6 tbsp unsalted butter
- 5 tbsp extra-virgin olive oil
- 1/3 cup of fresh lemon juice
- 1/2 cup of chicken stock
- 1/4 cup of brined capers, rinsed
- 1/3 cup chopped of fresh parsley

Directions

1. Season the chicken with pepper and salt Dredge the flour with the chicken and shake off the excess.

2. Melt 2 tbsp of butter with 3 tbsp of olive oil in a large skillet over medium-high fire. Add 2 pieces of chicken and cook for 3 minutes when the butter and the oil begins to sizzle. Flip and cook on the other side for 3 minutes when the chicken is browned. Remove the tray and pass it. Melt a further 2 tablespoons of butter and add another 2 tablespoons of olive oil. Add the other 2 pieces of chicken and brown both sides in the

same way as the butter and oil starts to sizzle. Take the pan out of the heat and add the chicken to the bowl.

3. The lemon juice, stock and capers are integrated through the pan. Return to the stove, bring to a boil and scrape the brown bits out of the pan for extra spice. Seasoning Check. Give to the pan all the chicken and cook for 5 minutes. Remove the chicken from the pan. Add to the sauce the remaining 2 teaspoons of butter and whisk vigorously. Pour the sauce over the chicken and add the parsley to the garnish.

VEGETABLE RECIPES

20.GREEN FRITTERS

Prep:15 mins

Cook:15 mins

Ingredients

- 140ggratedcourgettes
- 3 medium eggs
- 85g finely chopped broccoli florets,
- small packroughly chopped dill
- 3 tbsp gluten-free flour or rice flour
- 2 tbsp sunflower oil , for frying

Method

To remove any remaining moisture, pinch the courgettes between your palms, or tip over a clean tea towel and curl it to squeeze out the moisture.

In a bowl, beat the eggs, add the broccoli, courgettes and much of the dill, and blend. Add the flour, blend and season again.

In a non-stick frying pan, heat the oil. Put the mixture into the pan with a large serving spoon, and add 2 more spoonfuls so that you have 3 fritters. Leave on a medium heat for 3-4 mins until one side is golden brown and solid enough for you to turn over, then flip over and leave on the other side to go golden. Repeat for 3 more fritters to make (there is no need to add any more oil to the pan after the first batch). Scatter to eat with the remaining dill to.

21.RADISH CHIPS

Prep Time:10 mins

Cook Time:10 mins

Total Time:20 mins

Ingredients

- Oil for deep frying preferably palm oil
- 16 oz radishes
- ½ tsp coarse salt kosher
- US Customary – Metric

Instructions

1. Heat 2 to 3 inches of oil to 325 °F in a deep fat fryer or a large saucepan.

2. Cut the radishes into very thin slices, using a mandolin slicer or a very sharp knife.

3. Place the radishes in a jar and cover them with water. Boiling blood. Boil for 4 to 5 minutes over high heat or until the radish is transparent and the skin lightens. Drain the slices of radish in a colander.

4. To stop splattering, slowly add the radish slices to the hot oil.

5. Fry the slices of radish in hot oil for 8 to 10 minutes or till they turn a dark golden brown colour.

6. On paper towels, rinse and season with salt.

notes

If you choose not to deep fry them, radish chips can be cooked in the oven. To roast, after boiling and draining, pat them dry with paper towels, then bake at 350°F until they turn brown and crisp. It's best to really finely cut the radishes.

Nutrition

Calories: 48 calories

22.GARLIC ROASTED CARROTS

prep time: 5 MINUTEScook time: 40 MINUTEStotal time: 45 MINUTES

INGREDIENTS

- 24 baby carrots, tops trimmed to 2 inches
- 2 tbsp olive oil
- 2 tbsp balsamic vinegar
- 5 cloves minced garlic
- 1 tsp dried thyme
- Kosher salt and freshly ground black pepper, as need
- 2 tbsp chopped parsley leaves

DIRECTIONS

1. Preheat the oven to 375° F. Oil a baking sheet thinly or brush with nonstick paint.

2. Layer the carrots on the prepared baking sheet in one single layer. Add olive oil, balsamic vinegar, garlic then thyme and, if necessary, season with salt and pepper. Toss softly to blend.

3. Place the mixture in the oven and cook for 35-40 minutes or until tender.

4. Serve right away, garnished, if needed, with parsley.

Nutrition Facts

Calories 59.5

23.QUICK ROASTED TOMATOES

Prep Time 5 minutes

Cook Time 40 minutes

Total Time 45 minutes Ingredients

Ingredients

- 4 pounds cocktail, roma, plum, or cherry tomatoes
- 2 tbsp extra virgin olive oil
- 6-8 cloves whole garlic
- 1/2 tsp kosher salt
- 1/2 tsp freshly ground black pepper
- 10 sprigs fresh herbs such as thyme, basil, parsley, or rosemary

Instructions

1. Preheat the furnace to 400 degrees F. Cover with aluminium foil over a rimmed baking sheet.

2. You should leave the tomatoes whole by using cherry or cocktail tomatoes. I stem the tomatoes first for the plum or romas, then slice them in half lengthwise. By softly pressing them out (if you feel like it), choose the seeds or remove them with a spoon.

3. Lay the tomatoes in a single layer on a baking sheet lined with foil, cut side up when cut in half. Roast at 400 ° F for 40-50 minutes or until the skin softens and begins to burst, for cocktail, roma, or plum tomatoes. Roast for 15-20 minutes in the case of cherry tomatoes.

4. For a basic pasta sauce, discard the herbs and strip, cut or substitute entire salads, beans, or rice; mash and spread on toasted crostini; or add the garlic and tomatoes to a blender and whiz until smooth.

24.GARLIC BREAD

PREP TIME:5 mins

COOK TIME:13 mins

TOTAL TIME:18 mins

SERVINGS:4 to 8 servings

Ingredients

- 1 16-ounce loaf of Italian bread
- 1/2 cup of unsalted butter, softened
- 2 large and minced cloves garlic smashed
- 1 heaping tbsp of freshly chopped parsley
- 1/4 cup of freshly grated Parmesan cheese 24

Method

1. METHOD 1: TOASTED GARLIC BREAD

2. Preheat oven to 350°F

3. Prepare the garlic bread

4. Cut the loaf in two, horizontally. Mix the sugar, garlic, and parsley together in a small bow.Layer the butter mixture over the two halves of the loaf.

5. lBread spread with garlic butter for homemade garlic bread

6. Heat in oven for 10 min

7. Place on a durable baking pan (one that can handle high temperatures, not a cookie sheet) and fire in a 350°F (175°C) oven for 10 minutes.

8. Sprinkle with Parmesan (optional) and broil

9. Remove pan from oven. Sprinkle Parmesan cheese over bread if you like. Return to oven on the top shelf.

10. Broil on high heat for 2-3 minutes before the sides of the bread begin to toast and the cheese (if you are using cheese) bursts. Monitor very cautiously as

11. broiling. The bread will quickly go from un-toasted to burnt.

12. Slice

13. Remove from oven, let cool a minute. Remove from pan and use a bread knife to cut into 1-inch thick slices. Serve instantly.

14. Homemade garlic bread sliced into slices.

25.PRINT THIS GARLIC RANCH PRETZELS RECIPE BELOW

Prep Time:5 mins

Cook Time:20 mins

Total Time:25 mins

Ingredients

- 1/2 cup of Oil
- 1 tsp Garlic Powder
- 1 packet Ranch Dressing Mix Or 2 Tbsp of your homemade mix
- 1 lb Bag of Pretzels

Instructions

1. In a big bowl combine the oil, garlic powder, and Ranch dressing blend. Mix well.
2. Stir in the whole bag of pretzels and stir to cover full.
3. Spread out onto a baking sheet.
4. Baked at 270 degrees Fahrenheit for 20 minutes.
5. Allow it to totally cool down and relax!

6. Using an airtight container to hold leftovers.

Recipe Notes

- From game days to holidays to after school treats, this is a recipe I still go back to.

Nutrition Facts

Calories 233Calories from Fat 90

26.THE BEST FRENCH BREAD PIZZA RECIPE

YIELD:Serves 3 to 4

ACTIVE TIME:30 minutes

TOTAL TIME:30 minutes

Ingredients

- 3 tbsp butter
- 4 tbspdividedextra-virgin olive oil
- 4 clovesfinely minced garlic,
- pinch red pepper flakes
- 1/2 tsp dried oregano
- 1/4 cup of minced fresh parsley or basil leavesor a mix
- salt Kosher
- 1 large loaf French or Italian bread about 18 inches long and 4 inches wide, split half lengthwise and crosswise
- 1 can crushed tomatoes
- 8 ounces freshly grated whole milk mozzarella cheese
- 2 ounces grated Parmigiano-reggiano

Directions

1. Adjust oven rack to upper place and preheat oven to 425°F. Heat butter and 3 tbsp olive oil in a medium saucepan over medium-low heat until butter is melted. Add the garlic, oregano, and pepper flakes and cook, stirring occasionally, until the garlic is tender. but not browned, around 2 minutes. Stir in half of parsley/basil and a large pinch of salt. Remove from heat.
2. 2. On a clean work surface, place bread cut-side-up. Using a rimmed baking sheet, press down on bread uniformly

until compressed to around 2/3rds of its original height. Place bread on top of the baking sheet that is rimmed. Using a pastry rub, brush half of garlic/butter/oil mixture uniformly over cut surfaces of bread, making sure to get plenty of bits of garlic and aromatics. Set back.

3. Add tomatoes to remaining garlic/butter/oil mixture in pan, stir to blend, raise heat to low, bring to a simmer, then reduce heat to sustain a bare simmer. Cook for about 15 minutes, stirring occasionally, until rich and reduced.Season as need with salt.

4. as sauce cooks, scatter 1/4 of mozzarella thinly over surface of bread and transfer to oven. Cook until cheese is scarcely melted, about 8 minutes. Remove from oven and set aside before sauce is cooked.

5. Spread sauce thinly over bread, then spread leftover mozzarella on top of sauce. Transfer to oven and bake until cheese is melted and just beginning to brown, about 10 minutes. Remove from the oven and sprinkle easily with Parmigiano-reggiano, remaining parsley/basil, and remaining tbsp extra-virgin olive oil. Allow to cool slightly and serve.

27.SMOKY CHICKPEAS WITH SPINACH

Prep Time:3 mins

Cook Time:7 mins

Total Time:10 mins

Ingredients

- 1½ tbsp extra virgin olive oil
- 2 minced garlic cloves
- 1 tsp smoked paprika
- ½ tsp ground turmeric
- 2 cups of cooked chickpeas
- 6 cups of fresh spinach
- 2 tbsp water or vegetable broth

Instructions

1. Heat the olive oil over medium heat in a skillet. Add the ginger, turmeric, and smoked paprika. Stir. Heat the mixture of spices and oil for 1-2 minutes, until fragrant.
2. Add chickpeas and swirl to cover with the oil and spice mixture. Add spinach and water. Cook over medium heat before the spinach wilts. If ordered, add salt and pepper.. Serve!

Notes

- Cook the spices in the olive oil. This helps unlock the aromatic oils and heighten the taste in this recipe.
- Don't crowd the pan. If you add too much too a tiny skillet the chickpeas would be soft and not have the lovely caramelized taste.

- Using more lettuce than you think is comfortable. It will shrink so feel free to use a whole bunch or bag of spinach.

Nutrition

Calories: 355kcal

28.HOW TO TOAST MACADAMIA NUTS

READY IN: 15mins

SERVES: 4-6

YIELD: 100 grams

UNITS: US

INGREDIENTS

- 100
- g macadamia nuts
- parchment paper

DIRECTIONS

1. Preheat oven to 325 degrees Fahrenheit.
2. Cover baking sheet with parchment paper or aluminum foil (optional) (optional).
3. 3. For 10-12 minutes or until finely browned, toast the nuts.
4. PRINT RECIPE
5. Send a Recipe Correction.
6.

29.CRISPY FRIED SPINACH

PREP TIME:10 minutes

COOK TIME:5 minutes

TOTAL TIME:15 minutes

INGREDIENTS

- 250g fresh spinach
- oil for deep fryingVegetable
- Salt as need

INSTRUCTIONS

1. Dust the spinach leaves and dry them.
2. 2. Remove and shred with a sharp knife and stems and shred. You can see how I did this in the pictures above.
3. Heat the oil in a large pan. When a slice of spinach immediately sizzles when applied to the oil, you're ready to go.
4. Depending about how much you are making, you may need to cook the shredded spinach in batches.
5. When the spinach heats, it can turn a pair of shades darker. That is a pretty good sign that it is set.
6. Drain fried crispy spinach on paper towels. It should crisp right up once out of the liquid. Season with a little salt.

30.STUFFED GREEN PEPPERS

Level: Easy

Total: 2 hr (includes cooling time)

Active: 40 min

Yield: 6 servings

Ingredients

- Select All
- 6 medium green bell peppers, tops and seeds removed
- 2 tbsp vegetable oil
- 1 largefinely chopped onion
- Kosher salt
- 1 pound ground beef
- 2 largefinely chopped cloves garlic
- Freshly ground black pepper
- One 28-ounce can diced fire-roasted tomatoes
- 2 cups of cooked rice
- 1 cup ofroughly chopped
- loosely packed fresh parsley leaves,
- 1 1/2 cups of shredded mozzarella
- 1/2 cup of plain dry breadcrumbs
- 2 large lightly beaten eggs
- 4 tsp Worcestershire sauce

DIRECTIONS

1. bring to a high boil. Arrange the peppers in the steamer to shield the pot and cook the peppers by turning as desired, until they are very tender and pliable, around 25 minutes.

Remove the peppers with a slotted spoon, then drain upside-down on paper towels.

2. Put the oil, onions and a pinch of salt in a large skillet over medium heat, and fry, stirring periodically, until the onions are soft and translucent, around 8 minutes. Boost the heat to medium-high. Add the beef, garlic, 2 tsp salt and a few grinds of pepper, and cook, stirring and breaking the beef up, until browned and almost cooked through, about 5 minutes. Add the tomatoes and bring them to a boil, then remove them from the heat.Let it cool for at least 10 minutes in a skillet.Transfer to a big bowl and stir in the barley, parsley, 1 cup of mozzarella and 1 cup of mozzarella.The mixture of breadcrumbs, eggs and Worcestershire and match.

3. 3. In a 9-by-13 inch baking dish, stand up the peppers. If they tip over, hack away a little of the bottoms (without going into the pepper) to make a flat top.

4. 4. Fill and pack the peppers generously with the meat-rice mixture. Cover with the remaining 1/2 cup of mozzarella. To support steam, add just enough water to the pan to cover the bottom the peppers. Cover loosely with foil, then bake until tender and the peppers are tender. filling is heated through, about 30 minutes. Remove the foil, and proceed to bake for 10 minutes mo.

My Private Notes

- Categories:BellPeppersBeefTomatoRiceRecipesAppetizer

- More From: Autumn Weeknight Dinners

31.BAKED ZUCCHINI FRIES

yield: 6 SERVINGSprep time: 15 MINUTEScook time: 20 MINUTEStotal time: 35 MINUTES

INGREDIENTS:

- 1 cup of Panko*
- 1/2 cup of freshly grated Parmesan cheese
- 1 tsp Italian seasoning
- Kosher salt and freshly ground black pepper, as need
- 4 zucchini, quartered lengthwise
- 1/2 cup of all-purpose flour
- 2 large beaten eggs
- 2 tbsp chopped fresh parsley leaves

DIRECTIONS:

1. Preheat oven to 425 degrees F. Cover a cooling rack with nonstick spray and place on a baking sheet; set aside.
2. In a large bowl, mix Panko, Parmesan and Italian seasoning; Season with salt and pepper, if needed. Set back.
3. Function in batches, dredge zucchini in flour, dip into eggs, then dredge in Panko mixture, pressing to coat.
4. Place zucchini onto lined baking sheet. Place into oven and bake for 20-22 minutes.
5. Serve promptly, garnished with parsley, if desired.

NOTES:

- Panko is a Japanese-style breadcrumb which can be purchased in the Asian portion of your nearest grocery store.

Nutrition Facts

Calories 135.4Calories from Fat 40.5

32.SALT AND VINEGAR CHICKEN WINGS

Prep Time10 mins

Cook Time1 hr 10 mins

Total Time1 hr 20 mins

Ingredients

- Wings:
- 2 pounds Chicken Wings - separated into drumettes and flats
- 2 ½ tsp Baking Powder - DO NOT use baking soda!
- 1/2 tsp Kosher Salt
- Sauce
- 1/2 Cup of White Distilled Vinegar
- 6 TBS Malt Vinegar -
- 2 TBS Flaky Sea Salt - + more for garnishing
- 2 1/4 tsp Dry Ranch Mix
- 1 tsp Granulated Sugar
- ¼ tsp Garlic Powder
- Optional for Garnish: Sliced Chives or Scallions, Flaky Sea Salt

Instructions

1. Make salt and vinegar sauce: In a small container or container with a close-fitting lid, combine all the sauce ingredients together. Shake vigorously to combine all the materials fully, ensuring that the salt and sugar are dissolved.

2. Marinate Chicken Wings: In a big zip-closure bag, place the chicken wings. Over the wings, add half the salt and vinegar sauce. Shake and close the bag to coat the wings. Transfer to the refrigerator and allow to marinate before overnight or for at least 3 hours.

3. Preheat oven: Set one oven rack in the lower third position and one rack in the oven in the upper third position. Preheat the oven to 250°F. For speedy clean-up, cover a large rimmed baking sheet with aluminum foil. Place the insert on a wire rack on top of the baking sheet. To prevent the wings from sticking, coat the rack with non-stick cooking spray.

4. Clean the wings and toss with the baking powder: remove the chicken wings from the marinade and shake thoroughly off the wings with additional marinade. Remove the marinade. Transfer wings lined with paper towels to a clean work surface. Pat the wings absolutely dry. To a large zip-closure bag, shift the dried wings. To the shell, add the baking powder and kosher salt. To sufficiently cover the wings, seal and shake the bag vigorously. In a single layer, transfer the wings SKIN SIDE UP to the wire rack baking sheet.

5. Low Heat Cook Chicken Wings: Bake the chicken wings in the oven for 30 minutes on the LOWER shelf.

6. High Heat Cook Chicken Wings: Transfer the wings to the UPPER shelf and increase the temperature of the oven to 425 F. For an additional 20 minutes, bake. Take the oven wings and flip them over. Return to the oven and finish roasting for 20 minutes, or the skin is crispy and the chicken is cooked through until the wings are golden brown.

7. Toss and serve the wings: Remove the wings from the oven and place them in a large mixing bowl. Over the wings, pour the remaining salt and vinegar sauce. To coat, throw good. Serve promptly and enjoy yourself!

Notes

- To split chicken wings into drumettes and flats: cut wing tips with a sharp chef's knife, or kitchen shears, from chicken wings at the joint. Detach chicken drumettes from flats by cutting through the joint between the two (save tips to make stock or discard). It is quick to locate the joint, bending the flat sideways from the wing, revealing the joint.
- The recipe for the cooking method for these wings is adapted from Cook's Illustrated and Recipetineats.com
- Nutritional knowledge relies on 4 servings which is a preliminary estimate.

Nutrition

Calories: 293kcal

33.SALSA AND CHIPS

Level: Easy

Total: 20 min

Prep: 20 min

Yield: about 2 cups of

Ingredients

- Deselect All
- 4 plum tomatoes,and roughly chopped cored
- 1/2 mediumfinely chopped onion
- 1minced jalapeno
- 1/4 cup of chopped fresh coriander
- Kosher salt and freshly ground black pepper, as need
- Kosher salt and freshly ground black pepper, as need
- Tortilla Chips, recipe follows
- Tortilla Chips
- Vegetable oil for frying
- Twelve 6-inch corn tortillas
- Fine salt

Directions

1. Combine the tomatoes, cabbage, jalapeño, and cilantro in a shallow bowl. With salt and pepper season. Cover and set aside for 1 hour with plastic wrap. With Tortilla Chips, eat.

2. Chips from Tortilla

3. Yield: between 4 and 6 servings

4. Pour the oil to a depth of about 2 inches into a large, heavy-bottomed pot. In the pot, place a deep-frying thermometer. Heat the oil to 360 degrees F over a medium heat.

5. Stack the tortillas, respectively, and then cut the pile into sixths to make chips.

6. Improve the heat to a huge one. Function in batches, fry the chips for about 2 minutes, turn them with a skimmer or slotted spoon, until golden brown. To drain, transfer the chips to a paper towel-lined pan using a slotted spoon. (Return the oil between batches to the correct temperature.) Cool and season with salt. Just serve.

My notes to Private

• Send a Message

HealthyChipsSalsaJalapenoRecipesTomatoAppetizerGlutenFreeCinco de MayoVegan Vegan Categories:

• More From: Global Flavors: Weeknights

34.APPLE CHIPS

Prep:15 mins

Cook:45 mins

Additional:30 mins

Total:1 hr 30 mins

Servings:6

Yield:6 servings

Ingredients

2 Golden Deliciousand thinly sliced apples, cored

1 ½ tsp white sugar

½ tsp ground cinnamon

Directions

1. Preheat oven to 225 degrees F (110 degrees C) (110 degrees C).
2. Arrange apples slices on a wire baking sheet.
3. Pour sugar and cinnamon together in a bowl; scatter over apple slices.
4. Bake in the preheated until apples are dry and edges curl up, 45 minutes to 1 hour. Using a metal spatula to transfer the apple chips to a wire rack before cooled and crispy.

Cook's Notes:

- Slice apples using the chopping blade of a food processor or a mandoline.
- If you like, flip apple slices halfway through baking and dust the other side with cinnamon sugar. Note: they would not feel crispy until they cool off.
- Health Facts
- Per Serving: 24 calories; protein 0.1g; carbohydrates 6.9g; sodium 0.9mg. Total Diet

35.WATERMELON MINT LIME JUICE

Prep Time:15 mins

Total Time:15 mins

Servings: –6

INGREDIENTS

- 5-6 cups of cubed seedless watermelon
- Juice of 2 limes
- Handful of mint leaves

INSTRUCTIONS

1. In a blender, place everything and blend until smooth.

2. Strain juice over a fine mesh sieve and a large bowl if necessary. Pressure it out until there is just juice in the bowl and the pulp leaves in the sieve.

3. Pour into pots and prepare for up to five days in the refrigerator.

36.THE BEST CHOCOLATE CHIP COOKIE RECIPE EVER

Prep Time10 minutes

Cook Time8 minutes

Total Time30 minutes

Servings36 cookies

Ingredients

- 1 cup of salted butter softened
- 1 cup of white sugar
- 1 cup of light brown sugar packed
- 2 tsp pure vanilla extract
- 2 large eggs
- 3 cups of all-purpose flour
- 1 tsp baking soda
- ½ tsp baking powder
- 1 tsp sea salt
- 2 cups of chocolate chips
- US Customary - Metric

Instructions

1. Preheat the oven to 375° F. Cover and set aside a baking pan with parchment paper.

2. Mix the rice, baking soda, cinnamon and baking powder in a separate bowl. Just set back.

3. Cream the butter and sugar together when combined.

4. Whisk in the vanilla and eggs until fluffy.

5. When combined, throw in the dry ingredients.

6. Add a bag of 12 oz of chocolate chips and mix well.

7. Roll 2-3 TBS of dough at a time into balls (depending on how large you want your cookies) and place them evenly spaced on your prepared cookie sheets. (Alternatively, create the cookies using a small cookie scoop).

8. Bake in the preheated oven for 8-10 minutes or so. Let them out, so they're only BARELY going to turn brown.

9. Before removing them from the cooling rack, let them rest on the baking pan for 2 minutes.

Oh. 10. Video-Video

Notes

• Doughy. This is the secret that makes these cookies so totally awesome! I beg you, please, do NOT over-bake!

• Butter. To make those cookies, I use Costco's Kirkland Brand Salted Butter. With equally excellent results, I have also used salted butter from Tillamook. Unsalted butter is going to be perfect as well. To ensure it's salted to your liking, I just suggest tasting the dough.

Any users have said that they feel the cookies are too spicy. Make sure the natural sea salt (not iodized table salt) is used (not iodized table salt). Start with 1/2 tsp salt and conform to your tastes if you are concerned about saltiness. I still make salted butter and 1 teaspoon of sea salt with it.

Estimated recipe specifics based on 36 cookies produced by this recipe - 2 TBS of dough a piece)

• All-purpose flour: Many readers have used all-purpose gluten-free flour with good results.

Nutrition

183kcal Calories:

****BREAF ****

37.HASHBROWN BREAKFAST CASSEROLE

PREP TIME20 minutes

COOK TIME55 minutes

TOTAL TIME1 hour 15 minutes

SERVINGS8 servings

Ingredients

- 20 ounces shredded hash browns thawed
- 1 pound sausage cooked, crumbled and drained
- ¼ cup offinely diced onion
- ½ red bell diced pepper
- ½ green bell diced pepper
- 8 eggs
- 1 can evaporated milk 12 ounces, or 1 ⅓ cups of milk
- ½ tsp Italian seasoning
- salt & pepper as need
- 2 cups of cheddar cheese

Instructions

1. Preheat oven to 350°F (if baking immediately) (if baking immediately).
2. Brown sausage and dump fat.
3. Combine eggs, evaporated milk, salt & pepper, and Italian seasoning in a bowl. Whisk until smooth.
4. Place aside ½ cup of cheese for the topping.
5. Place remaining ingredients in a 9x13 baking tray. Pour egg mixture over the mixture and finish with remaining cheese.
6. Cover and refrigerate overnight if necessary.
7. Bake 55-65 minutes or until baked through.

Recipe Notes

- Remove from the fridge 30 minutes before baking whether the casserole is refrigerated overnight.. It can need an additional 10-15 minutes cook time.
- Evaporated milk can be replaced for 1 1/3 cups of milk.

NUTRITION INFORMATION

Calories: 413

38.BROCCOLI AND CHEESE EGG MUFFINS

PREP TIME:5 mins

COOK TIME:30 mins

TOTAL TIME:30 mins

YIELD:4 SERVINGS

INGREDIENTS

- 4 cups of broccoli florets
- 4 whole large eggs
- 1 cup of egg whites
- 1/4 cup of reduced fat shredded cheddar, Sargento
- 1/4 cup of good grated cheese like pecorino romano
- 1 tsp olive oil
- salt and fresh pepper
- cooking spray

INSTRUCTIONS

1. Preheat oven to 350°.
2. Steam broccoli with a little water for around 6-7 minutes.
3. When broccoli is baked, crumble into smaller parts and add olive oil, salt and pepper. Mix well.
4. Spray a normal size non-stick cup ofcake tin with cooking spray and spoon broccoli mixture uniformly into 9 tins.
5. In a medium bowl, beat egg whites, eggs, grated cheese, salt and pepper.
6. Pour into the greased tins over broccoli to a little more than 3/4 finished.
7. Cover with grated cheddar and bake in the oven until cooked, about 20 minutes. Serve instantly.

8. Wrap some leftovers in plastic wrap and store in the refrigerator to enjoy throughout the week.

39.COPYCAT OVEN-BAKED STARBUCKS EGG BITES

Prep Time: 15 minutesCook Time: 1 hourTotal Time: 1 hour 15 minutes Servings: 12 egg bit

Ingredients

- Bacon and Gruyere
- 1 tbsp olive oil
- 16 eggs, whisked
- 1 cup of bacon
- 1 cup of gruyere cheese
- Egg White and Red Pepper
- 1 tbsp olive oil
- 4 cups of egg whites
- 1 cup ofdiced roasted red peppers
- 1 cupfinely chopped of spinach,
- 1 cup ofmonterey jack cheese,

Instructions

1. Note: Select one version for this recipe; cut each of the ingredients in half if you want to do both versions (like in the video) Preheat the oven to 325 F. Fill halfway with warm water with a 9x11 baking dish, then place a greased 12-count silicone egg tray overtop.

2. Divide the toppings of choice and cheese into egg cups, then fill with eggs or egg whites the rest of the way. Bake for 60 minutes in the oven or until the eggs are ready.

3. When cold, cut egg bites from the molds and serve and enjoy!

Notes

- Nutrition info is for one regular egg bite; every of the egg white bites is 52 calories (1.25 g carbs, 1.98 g fat, 6.75 g of protein) (1.25 g carbs, 1.98 g fat, 6.75 g of protein)

Nutrition:

Calories: 178kcal .

40.VEGETABLE FRITTATA

prep Time10 mins

Cook Time15 mins

Total Time25 mins

Ingredients

- 6 eggs
- 1/4 cup of full fat yogurt optional
- 1 cup of shredded divided mozzarella cheese
- ¼ cup ofchopped red onions
- 1 cup of chopped mushrooms
- 8-10 stalks and chopped asparagus ends trimmed
- ¼ cup ofchopped cilantro
- ½ cup ofsliced cherry tomatoes

Instructions

1. Preheat the oven to degrees 425°.

2. Whisk the egg, milk, half the shredded mozzarella cheese and salt & pepper together; set aside the mixture.

3. In an oven safe pan or cast iron pan, heat the olive oil. Add the carrots, mushrooms and asparagus and steam for 3-5 minutes before softening the vegetables.

4. On top of the fried vegetables, pour the egg mixture on top. Place on top of the cherry sliced tomatoes and add the remaining cheese.

5. Bake in the preheated oven, uncovered, until the center is set and not jiggly, around 10-15 minutes.

Notes

Storage: Certain leftovers are kept in an air-tight bag. They will last up to 3 days in the refrigerator.

Freezing Instructions: The frittata can also be frozen for up to 3 months. To reheat, thaw overnight in the refrigerator and bake until baked in a 350 ° F oven. In the microwave, however, I would stop reheating because it will let out too much moisture from the vegetables to get a rubbery feeling.

Substitutes: Follow the formula as is, for the best results. Here, however, are some common replacements that in this recipe will work well.

• Yogurt is largely optional. You should use ricotta or sour cream instead of milk for a more smooth flavor. You may use milk that is either normal, or milk dependent on plants.

For some, you can replace the vegetables.

Feel free to swap the cheese for some other cheese you would like.

Nutrition: Please notice that an estimate based on an online nutrition calculator is the nutrition label provided. It will vary based on the exact ingredients you are using. This content should not be considered a replacement for advice by a professional nutritionist. For one meal, which is about 1 1/2 eggs + the vegetables I use, the nutrient advantage is. Using other vegetables will change the specifics of your diet.

Nutrition

Calories: 216kcal

41.AVOCADO TAQUITOS RECIPE

Prep Time5 minutes

Cook Time6 minutes

Total Time11 minutes

Servings4

Ingredients

- 6-8 corn tortillas
- 2-3 medium avocados
- 3/4 cup of Mexican blend cheese
- salt and pepper as need

Instructions

1. dd oil to a frying pan and place on medium heat.
2. Add avocados, cheese, salt and pepper to a bow and blend well. Spoon about ¼ cup of into the center of every corn tortilla. Roll up and place seam-side down in oil.
3. 3. Cook until golden on both sides Place on paper towel-lined plate to allow excess oil to drip off.
4. Serve warm and ENJOY!

42. TURKEY BROCCOLI EGG FRITTATA MUFFINS

Prep Time: 15 minutes Cook Time: 30 minutes Yield: 12 egg muffins

INGREDIENTS

- 1 pound ground turkey
- 12 eggs
- 1 cup of broccoli florets
- 1 cup of whole milk
- 1 tsp salt
- 1 tsp pepper

INSTRUCTIONS

1. Preheat oven to 350 degrees.
2. Brown Ground Turkey in a medium-sized skillet. Drain excess grease if needed and add turkey to mixing bowl.
3. Add broccoli and add about an inch of water to the bottom of the bowl in a medium-sized secure microwave bowl. Cover with plastic wrap and steam for 2-3 minutes. Carefully remove from microwave and add to broad mixing bowl.
4. Let broccoli and turkey cool for just a few minutes.
5. Add eggs, milk, salt and pepper to the mixing bowl. Whisk foods together.
6. Using a glass measuring cup of with a spout to scoop ingredients and pour into a greased muffin tin.

7. Bake until the eggs are ready, for 30-34 minutes..

8. Enjoy right away or allow to cool fully before storing.

43.SAUSAGE POTATO HASH

Prep: 10 mins

Cook: 20 mins

Total: 30 mins

Serves: 4

INGREDIENTS

- 2 tbsp olive oil
- 3 large potatoes peeled and cubed
- 1/2 tsp salt or as need
- 1/4 tsp pepper or as need
- 1 smallchopped onion
- 3/4 lb Italian sausage mild, casings removed
- 1/2 red chopped bell pepper
- 1/2 green chopped bell pepper
- 3 clovesminced garlic
- 1/4 tsp red pepper flakes
- US CUSTOMARY – METRIC

INSTRUCTIONS

1. ium heat. Add the cubed potatoes, season with salt and pepper and simmer for 7 to 10 minutes, until they're about half way cooked through, stirring periodically.
2. Add the onion and roast for another 3 minutes, stirring occasionally.
3. Add the bacon, bell peppers, garlic and red pepper flakes to the pan and stir. Reduce the fire, and continue cooking

until potatoes are cooked through, another 10 minutes. You should also cover the pan, this will cook the potatoes a little quicker.

4. Taste for seasoning and change with salt and pepper if appropriate. Serve with fried eggs.

RECIPE NOTES

- an egg, but feel free to choose a spicy sausage for more of a kick.
- Potatoes: I used Yukon Gold potatoes in this recipe, but you can also use russet potatoes.
- Please bear in mind that nutritional information is a rough approximation and can vary greatly depending on items used.

Nutrition Information

Calories: 593kcal (30%)

44. BAKED OATMEAL II

Cook:40 mins

Total:50 mins

Servings:8

Ingredients

- 3 cups of rolled oats
- 1 cup of brown sugar
- 2 tsp ground cinnamon
- 2 tsp baking powder
- 1 tsp salt
- 1 cup of milk
- 2 eggs
- ½ cup of melted butter
- 2 tspextract vanilla
- ¾ cup of dried cranberries

Directions

1. Preheat the oven to 175 degrees Celsius (350 degrees F) (175 degrees C).

2. Combine the oatmeal, brown sugar, cinnamon, baking powder, and salt in a large bowl. Add the milk, eggs, melted butter and vanilla extract to the mixture. Add the dried cranberries. Spread into a baking dish measuring 9x13 inches.

3. Bake in a preheated oven for 40 minutes.

Nutrition Facts

393 calories; fat 15.3g

45.SPICY SWEET POTATO HASH

Prep:10 mins

Cook:15 mins

Total:25 mins

Servings:2

Ingredients

- 2 strips uncured chicken bacon
- 2 medium sweet potatoes, cubed
- 1 tbsp olive oil, or more as needed
- 1 largefinely chopped jalapeno pepper,
- 1 ½ tbsp BBQ sauce
- 1 tsp garlic powder
- 1 pinch ground dried chipotle pepper
- salt and ground black pepper as need

Directions

1. In a large skillet, position the bacon and cook over medium-high heat, rotating occasionally, until browned evenly, around 5 minutes. When cool enough to touch, drain on paper towels and crumble.

2. Place the cubed sweet potatoes in a microwave-safe bowl and microwave for 5 minutes on high power while the bacon heats up.

3. Over low fire, heat a broad skillet. Add the sweet potatoes, garlic powder, chipotle powder, cinnamon, and black pepper and add the olive oil. Cook for 5 to 7 minutes, until the potatoes are brown and crisp. Add bacon, jalapeno, and BBQ sauce, then simmer for 2 to 3 more minutes over low heat.

Notes

Microwave for up to 8 minutes while using regular potatoes and use a cover on your skillet to guarantee good browning and even heating.

Nutrition Facts

279 calories; fat 7g;

46.SPINACH-EGG BREAKFAST PIZZAS

Total Time

Prep: 20 min. Bake: 15 min

Ingredients

- Cornmeal
- 1 pound frozen pizza dough, thawed
- 1 tbsp+ additionaldivided extra virgin olive oil
- 5 to 6 ounces fresh baby spinach
- 1/3 cup of+ additionaldivided grated Parmesan cheese
- 3 tbsp sour cream
- 1 smallminced garlic clove
- 1/4 tsp sea salt
- 1/8 tsp+ additionaldivided coarsely ground pepper
- 4 large eggs

Directions

1. Preheat the furnace to 500 °. 15x10x1-in Line Two. Dust lightly with cornmeal; baking pans with parchment. Cut 4 bits of dough; spread and shape into 6-to-7-inches. Circles. Place them in pans.

2. Meanwhile, cook 1 tbsp of olive oil in a large skillet over medium-high heat. Add spinach; cook and stir before wilting begins, around 1-2 minutes. Combine the next 5 ingredients with spinach; scatter the mixture of spinach on each pizza. Leave a thin line along the edge of the elevated doughBake for 5 minutes on the lower shelf of the oven.

3. Remove from the oven; split every pizza with an egg in the middle. Return to the lower oven shelf and bake for 6-10 minutes until the egg whites are fixed, but the yolks are still runny. Drizzle olive oil over the pizzas; add extra parmesan and pepper to finish. Instantly serve.

Nutrition Facts

433 calories, 14g fat

47.EGG AND TOMATO SCRAMBLE

Total Time

Prep/Total Time: 15 min.

Makes

1 serving

Ingredients

- 1 plumpeeled and chopped tomato
- 1 tsp chopped fresh basil or 1/4 tsp dried basil
- 1 egg or egg substitute equivalent
- 1 tsp water
- 1 garlicminced clove
- 1 tsp olive oil, optional
- Salt and pepper as need, optional
- 1 slice bread, toasted

- Additional fresh basil, optional
- Buy Ingredients

Directions

1. Mix the tomato and basil in a shallow bowl; set aside. Then pound the egg, water and garlic in another bowl. Heat the oil in a small nonstick skillet if desired; add the mixture of eggs. Cook until the egg is almost set, then stir gently. Add the tomato mixture and, if desired, salt and pepper.

2. Cook and stir until the egg is totally set and the tomato is fully cooked. With bread, serve. If required, garnish it with basil.

Nutrition Facts

152 calories, 4g fat

48.INDIAN-STYLE CAULIFLOWER

PREP TIME

10 MINUTES

TOTAL TIME

25 MINUTES

8 SERVING

Ingredients

- 2tbsp olive oil
- 1tsp coriander seeds
- 1tsp cumin seeds
- 1tsp curry powder
- 1tsp turmeric powder
- 1large head cauliflower, cored, broken into 1-inch florets
- Kosher salt and freshly ground black pepper
- 1tsp finely grated peeled ginger
- 1tsp finely grated lime zest

Preparation

1. Preheat the oven to 450 degrees. In a large bowl blend the oil, coriander seeds cumin seeds curry and turmeric together. Using cauliflower to add

2. And with salt and pepper sesaon. To coat the cauliflower equally, toss. Arrange on a wide rimmed baking sheet in a single layer (scrape any extra seasoning from the bowl over the cauliflower) (scrape any extra seasoning from bowl over cauliflower). Roast for 10 to 15 minutes, until the cauliflower is

brown around the edges and crisp-tender. Transfer to a bowl and scatter over the ginger and lime zest. Serve at room temperature, or hotter.

49.ZUCCHINI SALAD

prep Time: 10 mins

Serves 4

Ingredients

- Lemon Vinaigrette, + 1/4 cup of minced shallot mixed in
- 3 small-medium zucchini
- 1/4 cup of toasted pine nuts
- 1 tbsp chopped chives
- Handful of basil
- Shaved Parmesan, optional
- Sea salt and freshly ground black pepper

Instructions

1. Using a vegetable peeler to peel the zucchini into thin strips. Place the zucchini in a large bowl, toss with drizzles of the seasoning, then transfer the zucchini to a platter.
2. Cover with the pine nuts, chives, basil, and a few shavings of Parmesan, if using. Drizzle with more dressing and season with salt and pepper, as required.

50.CINNAMON SUGAR BAKED PEVERYES

yield: 8 SERVINGS prep time: 5 MINUTES cook time: 10 MINUTES total time: 15 MINUTES

INGREDIENTS

- 4 large, ripe peveryes
- 3 tbsp butter
- 3 tbsp brown sugar
- 1/4 tsp cinnamon
- Pinch of nutmeg
- Pinch of cloves
- Pinch of salt
- Vanilla ice cream, for serving

INSTRUCTIONS

1. Preheat the oven to 375°C. Halve cut peveryes and cut pits. Arrange on a large pan or baking sheet.

2. Place a small slice of butter in the center of each mixture.

3. In a small bowl, combine the brown sugar, cinnamon, nutmeg, cloves and salt together. Sprinkle over peveryes of combination.

4. Bake for 8-12 minutes, or until golden and soft. Before serving, coat it with vanilla ice cream.

51.GARLIC EDAMAME

PREP TIME: 5 mins

COOK TIME: 10 mins

TOTAL TIME: 15 minutes

INGREDIENTS

- 1 bag frozen edamame
- 3 cloves garlic
- 2 tbsp olive oil
- coarse sea salt
- low sodium soy sauce

INSTRUCTIONS

1. Boil the edamame as instructed on box. Drain and set aside.
2. In a large skillet, heat 2 tbsp olive oil. Crush the 3 cloves of garlic, but leave them in 1 slice. Toss them into the skillet with the edamame (I did it in 2 batches) and saute until the outsides of the edamame are just browning.
3. Serve in a wide bowl with a bowl on the side for the edamame shells. Serve with low sodium soy sauce (regular works, but it's pretty heavy so you may want to cool it down a bit) and add a little wasabi paste if you have it.

52.PERFECTLY SALTED DIY ROASTED ALMONDS - SERIOUSLY THE BEST!

Prep Time :5 mins

Cook Time :15 mins

Total Time :20 mins

Ingredients

- 4½ cups of raw, whole almonds
- 1½ tbsp HOT water
- 1½ tsp sea salt
- 2 tbsp olive oil
- sea salt as need

Instructions

1. Preheat the oven to 375 degrees and use a large baking sheet to protect the silicone or parchment. In a large metal or ceramic mixing bowl place the raw almonds.

2. Stir 11/2 tsp of salt until nearly absorbed in the warm water that spills over the bowl's nuts then blend until all are covered.

3. Place the nuts in a single layer on the parchment-lined baking sheet.

4. Stir well and sprinkle on a single plate again and bake for 8 or so minutes. Depending to how the oven cooks for 6-8 minutes, the nuts should be nicely browned inside and out to test the doneness. When they start burning hard, keep an eye on them now, because you just don't want them to be undercooked because they're not going to be crisp.

5 .Once the nuts have stopped frying, return them to the large bowl and drizzle with olive oil. Throw out the sea salt right before spraying all the nuts before you leave. You can taste one but it's really sweet so be careful.

6. Cause the nuts to cool in the mug, or scatter them out in the pot to cool more easily. As the nuts cool they can absorb the oil.

7. Keep it at room temperature in an airtight jar.

Notes

- When the larger pan is larger, this almond volume suits on an 18x13-inch baking sheet in a single layer, eliminating the recipe to contain the nuts in a single layer.
- In the first few minutes of baking the nuts will become tender. Oil them up and let them sleep and they will be amazing and crisp!

Nutrition

196kca Fat: 17.8g Calories:

53.SWEET & SPICY ROASTED PARTY NUTS

Prep Time: 10 minutes

Cook Time: 25 minutes

Total Time: 35 minutes

INGREDIENTS

- 2 cups of whole almonds
- 2 cups of pecan or walnut halves
- 1 ½ cup of pepitas
- Optional but so good: 2 tbsp finely snipped
- 2 tbsp maple syrup
- 2 tbspmelted unsalted butter
- 1 ½ tsp kosher salt
- 1 tsp vanilla extract
- ¼ tsp cayenne pepper

INSTRUCTIONS

1. To 325 degrees Fahrenheit with preheat the oven. Line a large rimmed parchment paper baking sheet or a silicone baking mat so that the maple syrup doesn't get stuck to the pan (this is essential) (this is important). Fill the pan with the almonds pecans and pepitas and set it aside.

2. Combine the added rosemary (or any other extra seasonings), maple syrup melted butter cinnamon, vanilla, and cayenne (if using) in a small bowl (if you using).Stir until it is well mixed.

3. Spill the mixture over the nuts on the baking sheet that has been packed. Stir well, before finely coating all of the nuts. Spread the mixture around the pan in a single layer (the maple syrup will settle on the bottom of the pan, so that's all right).

4. Bake until almost no maple syrup remains on the parchment paper and the nuts are intensely golden 23 to 26 minutesstirring for the first 10 minutes and then every 5 minutes afterwards. (The maple syrup coating will harden when the pecans cool but it could be a little slippery right out of the oven.)

5. Withdraw the skillet from the oven and stir the nuts once more spreading them uniformly around the pan. Let them cool down for about 10 minutes then carefully separate any big clumps (this may or may not be necessary) while the nuts are still warm (this may or may not be necessary).

6. Let the pan cool fully with the nut mixture. They can be stored in a sealed bag at room temperature for up to 2 months.

NOTES

• Recipe adapted from my Naturally Sweetened Candied Pecans and Rosemary Roasted Nuts recipes.

- SALT NOTE: I like how the huge flakes of kosher salt make certain bites a little saltier than others but the weight of kosher salt varies a lot from brand to brand. I used a brand of Diamond Crystal salt. Use 1 tsp. if you're using Morton kosher salt. Using 34 tsp fine sea salt or standard table salt if using fine sea salt.
- Keep IT Gluten FREE/VEGAN: swap the butter for extra virgin olive oil.
- Shake IT UP: In this recipe feel free to mess around with the nuts; you'll need a total of 51/2 cups. Cashews work

all the way but don't ever crisp up. It will be sweet with hazelnuts. Instead of maple syrup I tried using honey but maple has a higher flavor and a more candied (not sticky) feel.

Nutrition Facts

Calories   202

Total Fat 18.4g

54.JALAPENO POPPERS

PREP TIME20 minutes

COOK TIME25 minutes

TOTAL TIME45 minutes

SERVINGS12 servings

Ingredients

- 12 jalapeno peppers
- 6 ounces cream cheese softened
- 1 tsp garlic powder
- 4 ounces sharpshredded cheddar
- 2 tbsp finely chopped chives
- ¼ cup of Panko bread crumbs
- 1 tbsp butter

Instructions

1. Preheat the boiler to 400 degrees F.

2. Wearing gloves, lengthwise slice the jalapenos in two.To scrape off the seeds and membranes using a small spoon.

3. In a bowl, add together the cream cheese, garlic powder, cheddar cheese and chives (if used) (if using).

4. Panko crumbs and melted butter are combined in a separate bowl.

5. Fill the jalapenos with blended cheese. A floor with crumbs.

6. Place on a baking sheet and bake until golden or 18-22 minutes.

7. Before eating, cool for 5-10 minutes.

NUTRITION INFORMATION

Calories: 104 Fat: 9g,

55.CRISPY BUFFALO CHICKEN WINGS

PREP:5 MINS

COOK:1 HR

TOTAL:1 HR 5 MINS

SERVES:8

INGREDIENTS

- 4 pounds chickenand flats wings cut into drumettes
- 1 tbsp aluminium free baking powder
- 1/2 tsp salt
- 2 tsp garlic powder
- Pinch of cracked pepper
- BUFFALO SAUCE:
- 1/4 cup of butter melted unsalted
- 1/2 cup of Frank's Original Red Hot Sauce
- 1-2 tbsp honey, white sugar or brown sugar

- BLUE CHEESE DIP:
- 1/2 cup of crumbled blue cheese softened
- 1/3 cup of sour cream
- 1/4 cup of mayonnaise
- 2 clovesminced garlic
- 1 tbsp lemon juice
- Pinch of salt
- Pinch pepper of cracked black
- TO SERVE
- Ranch dressing
- Blue cheese dressing for serving
- Celery sticks for serving

INSTRUCTIONS

1. Adjust the oven rack to the upper-middle location and preheat the oven to 450°F .To cover a rimmed baking sheet use aluminum foil and with place a heat-proof wire rack inside.

2. Typically Pat uses paper towels to clean chicken wings squeezing as much moisture as possible out. For them turn to a wide bowl.

3. In a shallow bowl combine the baking powder garlic powder salt and pepper stir well to balance and sprinkle the mixture over the wings. When evenly colored throw the wings into the baking powder mix.

4. Place the wings on the rack leaving approximately 1 inch for each wing.

5. Bake for 30 minutesturn and continue to cook once golden and crisp brown until brown and crispy brown.

6. When the wings are finished, combine the hot sauce, butter, and honey in a mixing bowl. Throw the wings into the sauce to cover them uniformly.

7. With ranch dressing or blue cheese sauce and celery sticks eat the wings directly.

NOTES

- Adopt measures 1-4 for crispier wings. Then refrigerate the exposed wings overnight. This implies that they are completely dried out.
- I tried both directions, and only found in the refrigerated wings a slightly crispier feel!
- Motivated by Intense Eats.

NUTRITION:

Calories: 411kcal,

56.ROAST STICKY CHICKEN-ROTISSERIE STYLE

Prep:10 mins

Cook:5 hrs

Additional:4 hrs

Total:9 hrs 10 mins

Servings:8

Ingredients

- 4 tsp salt
- 2 tsp paprika
- 1 tsp onion powder
- 1 tsp dried thyme
- 1 tsp white pepper
- ½ tsp cayenne pepper
- ½ tsp black pepper
- ½ tsp garlic powder
- 2 onions, quartered
- 4 pound whole chickens

Directions

1. Mix the cinnamon, paprika, onion powder, thyme, white pepper, black pepper, cayenne pepper, and garlic powder together in a shallow bowl. Remove and discard the chicken giblets. Rinse the chicken cavity with a paper towel and pat it dry. Rub inside and out with spice mixture for each chicken.

Through the cavity of every chicken, take 1 onion. Place the chickens with plastic wrap in a resealable bag or double cover. Refrigerate overnight, or for 4 to 6 hours at the very least.

2. Preheat the furnace to 120 degrees C (250 degrees F) (120 degrees C).

3. Place the chickens in a pan for roasting. Uncovered Bake With.

Nutrition Facts

586 calories;

; fat 34.3g

57.LEMON BUTTER CHICKEN

servings: 4

Prep :15 minutes

Cook :15 minutes

Ready in: 30 minutes

INGREDIENTS

- 4 chicken breasts, pounded to an even 1/3-inch thickness
- Salt and freshly ground black pepper
- 1/3 cup of all-purpose flour
- 1 Tbsp olive oil
- 4 Tbsp unsalted butter,divided sliced into 1 Tbsp pieces,
- 1 1/2 tsp minced garlic
- 1/2 cup of low-sodium chicken broth
- 3 Tbsp fresh lemon juice
- 1/2 tsp fresh lemon zest
- 1 1/2 Tbsp minced fresh parsley

Instructions

1. Season all the chicken sides with salt and pepper.
2. Place flour in a shallow dish then dredge all sides of chicken breasts in flour, one at a time.
3. 3. Over medium-high pressure, heat a 12-inch skille.
4. 4. Add olive oil and 1 tbsp of butter, melt butter and add a single layer of chicken breasts.
5. Sear until golden brown on bottom, about 4 - 5 minutes then flip and continue to cook until chicken registers 165 degrees in middle, about 4 - 5 minutes longer.
6. Transfer chicken to a plate thus leaving every little bit of excess oil in pan.
7. Reduce to medium flame, add garlic and saute 20 seconds, or until only lightly golden brown, then dump in chicken broth while scraping browned bits off.
8. Add in the lemon juice, bring the mixture to a boil, reduce the heat slightly and cook until the liquid is about half depleted, about 2 minutes.
9. Add in remaining 3 Tbsp butter and lemon zest, stir to melt butter.
10. Return chicken to skillet, spoon sauce over chicken and garnish with parsley. Serve warm.
11. Recipe source: inspired by my Lemon Butter Salmon.

Notes

- 2 (10 oz.) chicken breasts can be used instead. Then simply butterfly and halve the breasts (cut through the thickness of the 2 wide breasts), to produce 4.

Nutrition Facts

Calories 341

Fat 19g

58.LEMON PEPPER CHICKEN

4 SERVINGS

PREP TIME: 0 HOURS 15 MINS

TOTAL TIME: 0 HOURS 45 MINS

INGREDIENTS

- 1/2 c all-purpose flour
- 1 tbsp lemon pepper seasoning
- 1 tsp kosher salt
- 2divided lemons
- 1 lbhalved, boneless skinless chicken breasts
- 2 tbsp extra-virgin olive oil
- 2 cups Swanson Chicken Broth
- 2 tbsp. butter
- 2 minced cloves garlic
- Freshly chopped parsley for garnish

DIRECTIONS

1.APPLICATIONS FOR THE OVEN

2.Heat with the oven to 400 degrees F. Combine flour, lemon pepper, salt, and 1 lemon zest in a medium mixing bowl. Toss the chicken breasts in the flour mixture until fully coated. Round the remainder of the lemon into little rounds.

3. Heat the thermal oil in a large ovenproof skillet over medium-high heat. Cook the chicken breasts in a single layer until golden brown on the bottom, then flip and cook for another 5 minutes.

4. Add in the broth, garlic, and lemon slices into the skillet and bake until the chicken is cooked through and the sauce has reduced significantly, about 5 minutes.

5. Drizzle the sauce over the chicken and end with a sprinkling of parsley.

7. Blend rice, lemon pepper, salt, and 1 lemon zest in a medium mixing bowl. Toss the chicken breasts in the flour mixture until fully coated. Round the remainder of the lemon into little rounds.

8. In a big ovenproof pan, heat the oil over with medium-high heat. Cook the chicken breasts in a single layer for 5 minutes, or until golden on the bottom, before turning them.

9. Cook for 3 minutes, or until the chicken is cooked through and the sauce has reduced slightly, by adding the water, butter, garlic, and lemon slices to the pan.

10. Drizzle the sauce over the chicken and add the parsley on top.

59.HOW TO COOK A RIBEYE STEAK

yield: 3-4 SERVINGSprep time: 25 MINUTEScook time: 20 MINUTEStotal time: 45 MINUTES

INGREDIENTS:

- 1 bone-in ribeye steak, 2-inch-thick, at room temperature
- Kosher salt and freshly ground black pepper, as need
- 1 tbsp canola oil
- 3 tbsp unsalted butter
- 3 cloves garlic, smashed
- 3 sprigs fresh thyme
- 2 sprigs fresh rosemary

DIRECTIONS:

1. Pat all sides of the steak dry using paper towels; season generously with 1 1/4 tsp of salt and 1/2 tsp of pepper.

2. Over medium high pressure, heat a medium cast iron skillet until very hot, around 1-2 minutes; add canola oil.

3. In the center of the skillet, place the steak and cook, alternating every 2-3 minutes, until on both sides a dark crust has formed, around 12-14 minutes.

4. Lower the heat to low-medium hea. Push the steak to one side of the skillet; add the sugar, garlic, thyme, and rosemary to the other side of the skillet, tip the skillet toward the butter, and fry for about 30 seconds to 1 minute until the butter is foaming.

5. Working slowly, for 1-2 minutes, spoon butter over steak, turning over once, until an internal temperature of 120 degrees F for medium rare, or until maximum doneness is reverted. Leave to pause before slicing for 15 minutes.

6. Immediately serve

60.AIR FRYER CHICKEN WINGS

Prep Time: 4 minutes

Cook Time: 16 minutes

Total Time: 20 minutes

Ingredients

- 1 lb chicken wings split into flats and drummettes
- 1 Tbsp oil olive
- 2 tspsalt garlic
- 1 tsp lemon pepper

Instructions

1. Vigorously pat the dried chicken wings with paper towels and place them in a mixing bowl.

2. Coat 2 tsp of garlic salt with 1 tsp of lemon pepper and spray with 1 tbsp of oil. To clean the seasoning fairly, toss.

Place on a randomly spaced air frying basket and fry for 8 minutes per hand or a total of 16 minutes at 400 F or until chicken wings are crisp and golden brown on the outside.

Notes

If the formula is doubled, the air is fried or the wings are tossed for 18-22 minutes until the skin is halfway crisp. Depending on your air fryer basket's surface area, baking time can vary.

Nutrition Facts:

168 Calories,13g fat

61.SCALLOPS WITH DILL SAUCE

Prep:20 mins

Broil:8 mins

Servings:4

Ingredients

- 1 pound fresh or frozen sea scallops
- 3 tbspmelted butter,
- ¼ tsp black pepper
- ⅛ tsp paprika
- ⅔ cup of mayonnaise
- 1 tbsp finely chopped onion
- 2 tsp lemon juice
- 1 ½ tsp snipped fresh dillweed or 1/2 tsp dried dillweed
- Lemon wedges

Directions

1. Thaw scallops, if frozen. Rinse scallops; pat dry with paper towels. Halve some big scallops. Thread scallops onto four 8- to 10-inch skewers, leaving a 1/4-inch gap between bits. Preheat broiler. Place skewers on the greased unheated rack of a broiler tray.
2. Instructions Checklist
3. In a small bowl stir together sugar, pepper, and paprika. Brush half the dough over the scallops.Broil for 8 to 10 minutes or about 4 inches from the heat or broil for 8 to 10 minutes or until scallops are opaque, rotating and scraping with the remaining melted butter mixture halfway through broiling.
4. Instructions Checklist

5. Meanwhile, for tartar sauce, in a small bowl stir together mayonnaise, cabbage, lemon juice, and dillweed. Serve scallops with tartar sauce and, if desired, lemon wedges.
    6.Instructions Checklist
6. Makes 4 kabobs.

Nutrition Facts

451 calories; total fat 39g;

62.CHICKEN CACCIATORE

PREP:10 MINS

COOK:40 MINS

TOTAL:50 MINS

- ## *INGREDIENTS*

- 6 bone-in skinless chicken thighs
- Salt and pepper, to season
- 1 medium , diced onion
- 2 tbsp minced garlic
- 1 small yellow diced bell pepper
- 1 small reddiced bell pepper
- 1 largepeeled and sliced carrot
- 10 ozsliced mushrooms
- 1/2 cup of pitted black olives
- 8 sprigs thyme
- 2 tbspevery freshly chopped parsley and basil + more to garnish
- 1 tsp dried oregano
- 150 ml red wine
- 28 oz crushed tomatoes

- 2 tbsp tomato paste
- 7 ozRoma tomatoes, halved
- 1/2 tsp red pepper flakes

INSTRUCTIONS

7. With salt and pepper, season the chicken with.
8. With 2 teaspoons of oil, heat a large cast iron skillet. Sear the chicken on both sides once golden, 3-4 minutes on each side. Remove from the skillet and set aside.
9. . Add leftover oil to the pan. Sauté the onion for 3-4 minutes or so before it is translucent. Add the garlic and boil until it's fragrant for about 30 seconds. Add the peppers, onions, herbs and mushrooms; roast till the vegetables are tender for 5 minutes.
10. . Pour the wine onto the skillet's rim, grinding the browned bits off. Cook for about 2 minutes or so, before the wine decreases.
11. . Add crushed tomatoes, chilled flakes, tomato paste, and Roma tomatoes. Season with salt and pepper to your liking Return the chicken components to the skillet and start cooking as instructed below over the stove top OR in the oven.
12. . FOR FOR STOVE TOP:
13. . Combine all the ingredients together; cover with a seal, decrease the heat, and allow to boil for 40 minutes or until the bone falls off the beef (stirring occasionally). Add the olives, then simmer for 10 more minutes. Garnish it with parsley and serve promptly.
14. FOR the furnace: 14.
15. . Transfer the sealed skillet to a preheated oven at 375 ° F (190 ° C) and steam for 50 minutes. Remove the lid, add the olives and cook until the chicken is crispy and bone-free and the sauce is reduced for an additional 20 minutes.

NOTES

- FOR THIS Recipe FOR THE SLOW COOKER USE

• If the sauce is too weak for your needs, add 2 tbsp of additional tomato paste as it thickens to boil. AHEAD TO Prepare: This chicken cacciatore can be cooked, cooled, wrapped and chilled up to 1 day in advance. Over low-medium heat, rewarm. TO Hot the chilled cacciatore and pass it to the freezer in an air tight bag. The day before serving, in the morning, thaw it out and get it to room temperature. Transfer to a skillet/pan and reheat until cooked through, over low-medium heat.

NUTRITION

Calories: 310kcal Saturated Fat: 2g

63.CHICKEN CURRY

Prep Time15 mins

Cook Time45 mins

Total Time1 hr

Ingredients

- 2 mediumand quartered potatoes peeled
- ¼ cup ofoil canola
- 2 largeand cubed carrots peeled
- ½ greeninto cubes bell pepper coredseeded and cut
- ½ red bell pepperinto cubes coredseeded and cut
- 3 clovespeeled and minced garlic
- 1 thumb-sizeandpeeled julienned ginger
- 1 bone-in chickencut intopieces serving
- 1 tbspsauce fish

- 1 cupmilk of coconut
- 1watercup of
- 2 tbsppowder curry
- salt and pepper as need

Instructions

. Boil or until the potatoes are soft and well browned for around 2 to 3 minutes. Take it out of the pan and wipe it with wax on the towels.

2. For 1 to 2 minutes or so, introduce and cook the carrots. Take it out of the pan and wipe it with wax on the towels.

3. With the exception of around 1 tbsp remove the excess oil from the skillet. Add a few bell peppers and simmer for 30 to 40 seconds or so. Remove the pan from the fire and set it aside.

4. Substitute the onions with garlic and ginger and boil until softened.

5. Add the chicken and simmer until lightly browned, stirring occasionally.

6. Add fish sauce and continue to cook for 1 minute or so.

7. Add water and coconut milk. On top of any scum that can float, carry it to a boil and skim.

8. Lower the flame, cover, and roast for 20 to 30 minutes or until the chicken is cooked.

9. Add the carrots and potatoes and simmer for about 3 to 5 minutes or until tender.

10. To blend add the curry powder and stir. Keep boiling for another 2 to 3 minutes, or before the sauce starts to thicken.

11. As needed, season with salt and pepper.

12. Add the bell peppers and cook until soft yet crisp, or around 1 minute. Get wet served it.

Nutrition

Calories: 569kcal Fat: 45g

64.POT ROAST WITH VEGETABLES

Prep:20 mins

Cook:5 hrs 35 mins

Additional:10 mins

Total:6 hrs 5 mins

Servings:6

Ingredients

- 1 tbsp vegetable oil
- 1 pound boneless beef chuck roast
- salt and ground black pepper as need
- 1 largefinely chopped onion
- 1 clove garlic, chopped, or as need
- 2 ½ cups of beef stock
- 1 (16 ounce) can diced tomatoes
- ¼ cup of red wine vinegar
- 1 tbsp brown sugar
- 2 bay leaves
- ¾ pound carrots, cut diagonally into 1-inch-thick slices
- 1 pound small red potatoes, quartered lengthwise

- 1 jar mushrooms, or more as need
- 1 ½ tbsp cornstarch
- 1 ½ tbsp cold water
- 1 pinch celery salt, or as need
- 1 pinch dried basil, or as need
- 1 pinch dried thyme, or as need

Directions

1. Preheat the boiler to 150 degrees C (300 degrees F) (150 degrees C).

2. Over medium heat, heat vegetable oil in a huge, heavy pot or cast-iron Dutch oven. Brown chuck roast completely, 5 to 8 minutes per hand, in hot oil; season with salt and black pepper and transfer to a bowl. Pot reserve crude.

3. Cook and mix the onion and garlic in the oil for about 15 minutes until the onions are golden. Stir in onions and garlic with beef stock, tomatoes, red wine vinegar, brown sugar, and Leaves of the bay To a boil, bring the chuck roast and place in the mixture. Pot cover.

4. Roast in the preheated oven for 4 to 4 1/2 hours until the beef is very tender. Scatter slices of carrot around the beef and carry over medium heat to a boil; return for 30 more minutes to the oven. Distribute the potatoes around the beef and vegetables, bring to a boil over medium heat again, and bake for about 30 more minutes until the potatoes are tender.

5. Transfer beef to a serving bowl, cover it loosely with an aluminum foil tent, and set aside for 10 minutes to rest.

6. Stir mushrooms into pan drippings; over low heat, bring to a boil. In a shallow bowl, whisk the cornstarch in cold water and incorporate into the drippings. Use celery salt, basil, and thyme

to season. Simmer for about 5 minutes before it thickens. Remove the bay leaves and dispose them. Serving slices of beef on a tray surrounded by vegetables. Blend the gravy over the steak.

Nutrition Facts

567 calories fat 32.8g

65.HAMBURGER SOUP

PREP TIME10 minutes

COOK TIME25 minutes

TOTAL TIME35 minutes

SERVINGS8 esrvings

Ingredients

- 1 pound lean ground beef
- 1 diced onion
- 2 cloves minced garlic
- 2 medium peeled and diced potatoes
- 3 ½ cups of beef broth
- 28 ounces diced tomatoes with juice
- 1 can condensed tomato soup
- 2 tsp Worcestershire sauce
- 1 tsp Italian seasoning
- 1 bay leaf
- salt and pepper as need
- 3 cups of mixed vegetables fresh or frozen

Instructions

1. Black cabbage, ground beef and garlic until no pink remains. Drain some fat.
2. Add potatoes, broth, onions, tomato soup, Worcestershire sauce, spices and bay leaves. Simmer covered 10 minutes.
3. Stir in vegetables. Simmer for 15-20 minutes or until tender potatoes are available.

NUTRITION INFORMATION

Calories: 245Fat: 9g,

66.SESAME CHICKEN

Prep Time20 minutes

Cook Time20 minutes

Total Time40 minutes

Servings 6

INGREDIENTS

- For the chicken
- 1 1/2 lbs boneless skinless chicken breasts cut into 1 inch pieces
- 2beaten eggs
- salt and pepper as need
- 1/2 cup ofall purpose flour
- 1/2 cup of cornstarch
- oil for frying
- For the sauce
- 1 tsp vegetable oil
- 1 tsp minced fresh garlic
- 1/4 cup of honey

- 1/3 cup of soy sauce
- 1/2 cup of ketchup
- 3 tbsp brown sugar
- 2 tbsp rice vinegar
- 1 tbsp toasted sesame oil
- 2 tsp cornstarch
- 2 tbsp sesame seeds
- 2 tbsp sliced green onions

INSTRUCTIONS

. Smash the bowl with the egg, salt and pepper. 2. Stir to mix 2. In a small bowl or on a plate, place the flour and 1/2 cup cornstarch. To mix, stir.

3. In the egg mixture, dip each piece of the chicken, then into the flour. With the entire chicken, repeat the process.

4. Heat 3 inches of oil to 350 degrees F in a deep bathroom sink.

5. To the pan, add 7-8 chicken pieces. Cook for 5 minutes. With the remaining chicken, repeat the surgical process with.

6. Use paper towels to drain chicken to

7. Combine the butter, soy sauce, ketchup, brown sugar, sesame oil, rice vinegar and 2 tsp. cornstarch into a cup after the chicken is fried.

8. In a wide pan, heat the TSP of oil on a low heat. Add the garlic and allow it to boil for 30 seconds. Add the combination of honey sauce and get it to a boil. Cook for 3-4 minutes,

9. To the pan, add the fried chicken and spray with the sauce and toss. Sprinkle with green onions and sesame seeds, then eat.

NOTES

- The sauce can be prepared up to two days before you decide to eat it.

NUTRITION

Calories: 392kcaSaturated Fat: 6g

FISH DISHES

67.SPICY NEW ORLEANS SHRIMP

Prep: 5 mins Cook: 20 mins Marinating Time: 30 mins Total: 55 mins Serves: 2

INGREDIENTS

- 1 lb white tiger shrimp
- 2 tbspunsalted butter
- 2 tbsp oil olive
- 2 tbspsauce sweet chili

- 1Worcestershiretbsp
- 1 tsppowder chili
- 1 tsp liquid smoke
- 1 tsp smoked 1 tsp dried oregano
- 1 tsp sriracha hot sauce or tabasco
- 4 cloves minced garlic
- juice from 1/2 lemon
- salt and pepper as need
- 2 tbspchopped parsley
-

INSTRUCTIONS

1. Peel and devein the shrimp.
2. Add the rest of the ingredients to oven safe skillet, stir and let simmer for 5 to 10 minutes.
3. Remove skillet from the heat and let cool for a few minutes.
4. Add the shrimp and toss it around so that it's fully immersed in the sauce.
5. Cover with foil and refrigerate for at least 30 minutes to 4 hours.
6. Preheat oven to 400 degrees.
7. Bake shrimp for 10 to 15 minutes.
8. Serve immediately with crusty French bread and drizzle with extra lemon juice if requested.

RECIPE NOTES

- This recipe will last in an airtight bag for 3-4 days in the refrigerator, so feel free to prepare it in advanceWith this recipe, you can freeze shrimp in an airtight jar for up to 3 months. Only allow the dish to thaw in the fridge overnight before eating.
- Please note that dietary data is an approximate estimate and can differ considerably based on the products used.

Nutrition Information:

Calories: 443kcal

Fat: 28g A

68.LOBSTER TAIL FOIL PACKS WITH LEMON CHIVE BUTTER

SERVINGS:4

PREP TIME:10 min

COOK TIME:20 min

DURATION:30 min

Ingredients

- 1 lemondivided zested and juiced
- 1/4 cup of organic unsalted butter, room temperature
- 2 tbsp chopped fresh chives
- 1/8 tsp sea salt
- 1/4 tsp ground black pepper
- 1/8 tsp ground cayenne pepper
- 4 6-oz fresh or frozen shell-on lobster tails, thawed
- 12 baby potatoes, halved
- 2 ears corn, husked and cut into quarters
- 2 red bell peppers, quartered
- 1/2 cup of low-sodium chicken broth

Preparation

1. Heat a barbecue to big. In a shallow bowl, mix lemon zest, sugar, chives, salt, pepper and cayenne.
2. Arrange 4 12-inch-long double layers of heavy-duty foil on a work board. Use kitchen shears, cut through membrane on underside of any lobster tail to reveal meat. Take 1 lobster tail in middle of any stack of foil. Cover with potatoes, beans, bell peppers, broth, lemon juice and butter mixture, separating equally. Bring short edges of

every stack of foil together, then fold inward a few times around every long edge to seal packages.

3. heat on 1 side of the grill to mild. Place packets on low heat, close lid and grill until lobster meat is firm and opaque and vegetables are tender, 20 to 25 minutes.

Nutrition Information

Calories380

Fat Content14 g

69.SESAME SHRIMP

Prep Time:5 minutes

Cook Time:15 minutes

Total Time:20 minutes

Servings:4

INGREDIENTS

- 1 14 ounce box Gorton's Popcorn Shrimp
- 2 tbsp soy sauce
- 1/4 cup of ketchup
- 2 tbsp honey
- 2 tsp toasted sesame oil
- 2 tsp corn starch
- 1 tbsp sesame seeds
- 2 tbspsliced green onions

INSTRUCTIONS

1. Bake your shrimp popcorn according to the box instructions.

2. Make the sauce while the shrimp is in the oven. Combine the soy sauce, ketchup, honey and sesame oil in a small saucepan; bring to a boil.

3. Blend 1/4 cup of cold water with the cornstarch and whisk until smooth. Dump the cornstarch mixture slowly, whisking constantly, into the sauce. Bring it to a boil with the sauce. Cook until just thickened, or for 1 minute.

4. Extract the shrimp from the oven .Drizzle the shrimp with the sauce over the shrimp and toss to cover equally. Sprinkle on top of the shrimp with the sesame seeds and green onions and eat.

NUTRITION:

Calories: 321kcal ,

70.STEAMED TROUT WITH MINT & DILL DRESSING

Prep:10 mins

Cook:25 mins

Serves: 2

Ingredients

- 120g potatoes halvednew
- 170g pack asparagustrimmed spears woody ends
- 1 ½ tsp vegetable bouillon up to 225ml with waterpowder made
- 80g finetrimmed green beans
- 80g frozen peas
- 2 skinless trout fillets

- 2 slices lemon
- For the dressing
- 4 tbsp bio yogurt
- 1 tsp cider vinegar
- ¼ tspmustardpowder English
- 1 tsp finelychopped mint
- 2tspdill chopped

Method

1. In a pan of boiling water place the fresh potatoes to cook until tender. Trim the asparagus in half to shorten the spears and slice the ends without the tips. To tip the bouillon use a large non-stick pan. Add the asparagus and beans then cover and simmer for 5 mins.

2. Add the peas to the plate then finish with the trout and lemon slices. Cover it again and cook for 5 mins longer before the fish flakes very quickly so its still juicy.

3. Meanwhile, with the yogurt combine the vinegar, mustard powder mint and dill. To the fish add 2-3 teaspoons of the cooking juices. Serve with the potatoes the veggie and all other pan juices. Place in cups cover with fish and herb dressing.

71.CAJUN SPICED SALMON

Prep:20 mins

Cook:5 mins

Serves: 2

Ingredients

- 2 salmon fillets , about 140g/5oz every
- juice 1 lime
- pinch chilli powder
- ½ tsp ground cumin
- ½ tsp smoked paprika
- ½ tsp ground coriander
- pinch of soft brown sugar
- drizzle of sunflower oil
- steamed rice , to serve
- For the salsa
- 1peeled and diced ripe avocado
- handful cherry tomatoes , quartered
- 2 spring slicedonions ,
- juice 1 lime
- splash of olive oil
- bunch of coriander , half roughly chopped, half picked into sprigs

Method

1. Place the salmon in a bowl, pour over the lime juice and leave the salmon to 'cure' for 5 mins. Meanwhile, blend all the spices along with the butter. Lift the salmon out of the lime juice and roll in the seasoning so it's fully coated.

2. Heat grill to high. Grease a baking sheet, then sit the salmon, flesh-side up, on the tray. Grill for 5 mins, until the salmon is cooked through and the sides are beginning to blacken. When the salmon is frying, gently mix all the salsa ingredients along with the finely chopped coriander. When the fish is fried, serve with the salsa, some rice and the coriander sprigs.

72.BAKED CATFISH WITH HERBS

Prep Time: 5 minutesCook Time: 20 minutesTotal Time: 25 minutes Servings: 4 servings

Ingredients

- 2 tblsp. mincedparsley fresh
- 1 tsp salt
- ¾ tsp. paprika
- ½ tsp. dried thyme
- ½ tsp. dried oregano
- ½ tsp. dried basil
- ½ tsp. ground black pepper
- 4 whole catfish fillets
- Juice of one lemon
- 2 tblsp. melted butter
- ¼ tsp. garlic powder
- Non-stick cooking spray

Instructions

1. To 350 degrees Fahrenheit preheat the oven.
2. Combine the parsley, salt, paprika, thyme, oregano, basil and pepper in a small bowl.
3. Sprinkle on both sides of catfish fillets.

4. In a 9x13 baking pan that has been coated with non-stick cooking spray, place the fillets.
5. Add the melted butter, lemon juice and garlic powder to a small bowl. Mix well to blend.
6. Drizzle the butter-lemon-garlic mixture over the fillets.
7. Bake uncovered for 15-20 minutes or before the fish flakes easily.

Notes

- —Recipe adapted from Taste of Home's Busy Family Recipes, Winter 2011.

Nutrition Information

Calories: 265kcal |Fat: 16g

73.SIMPLE RANCHY BREADED FISH FILLETS

Prep:15 mins

Cook:10 mins

Total:25 mins

Servings:4

Ingredients

- ¾ cup of Italian seasoned bread crumbs
- 1 package dry Ranch-style dressing mix
- 2 ½ tbsp vegetable oil
- 1 pound tilapia fillets
- 2 tsp butter

DirectionsInstructions

1. Place the bread crumbs in a bowl In a shallow dish, blend the dressing mix and oil to form a paste. Cover the paste with the tilapia fillets, then dredge them in the bread crumbs to lightly coat them.
2. Melt the butter in a pan over medium heat Place the fillets in the skillet, and cook 5 minutes on either hand, or until golden brown and easily flaked with a fork.

Nutrition Facts

Calories :310kcal

74.GARLIC BUTTER SHRIMP SCAMPI

PREP:5 MINS

COOK:5 MINS

TOTAL:10 MINS

SERVES:4

INGREDIENTS

- 2 Tbsp olive oil
- 4 tbsp butter
- 4-5 largeminced garlic cloves
- 1 1/4 pounds large shrimp prawns, shelled with tails on or off
- Salt and fresh ground black pepper as need
- 1/4 cup of dry white wine or broth
- 1/2 tsp crushed red pepper flakes or as need
- 2 tbsp lemon juice
- 1/4 cup of chopped parsley

INSTRUCTIONS

1. In a large pan or skillet, heat the olive oil and 2 tbsp of butter. Add the garlic and sauté until fragrant (30 seconds - 1 minute approximately) (about 30 seconds - 1 minute). Then add the shrimp, season as appropriate with salt and pepper and sauté on one side for 1-2 minutes (until it just begins to turn pink), then flip.

2. Pour in wine (or broth), add (if using) red pepper flakes (if using). Bring to a boil for 1-2 minutes or till about half of the wine is reduced and the shrimp is cooked (do not overcook the shrimp).

3. Add the remaining butter, lemon juice and parsley and quickly take off the oven.

4. Eat over cauliflower, broccoli, zucchini noodles, potatoes, pasta, garlic bread or steamed vegetables (cauliflower, broccoli, zucchini noodles).

NUTRITION

Calories: 291kcal Fat: 13g

75.ZESTY TILAPIA WITH MUSHROOMS

Prep:15 mins

Cook:10 mins

Additional:20 mins

Total:45 mins

Servings:4

Ingredients

- 1 ounce dried porcini mushrooms
- 2 tbsp butter
- 2 fillets tilapia, halved
- kosher salt as need
- ground black pepper as need
- 1 tbsp lemon zest
- 2 limes, juiced
- 2 greenchopped onions

Directions

1. In a small bowl, place the dried porcini mushrooms with enough warm water to cover them. 20 minutes to soak, or until rehydrated, then chop.

2. In a medium skillet over medium pressure, melt 1 tablespoon of butter. Place the tilapia and season with kosher salt and pepper in the skillet. Sprinkle 1/2 of the lemon zest with it. Cover the tilapia with half the lime juice and finish cooking for 5 minutes.

3. Flip the tilapia and season with pepper and kosher salt. Sprinkle with the remainder of the lemon zest, and add the remaining lime juice. Stir in the pan with the remaining cinnamon, green onions, and porcini mushrooms. Continue to cook for 5 minutes or before the fish flakes easily with a fork.

Nutrition Facts

146 calories; fat 6.9g

76.CRISPY SOUTHERN FRIED CATFISH

Prep Time5 minutes

Cook Time10 minutes

Total Time15 minutes

Servings4 servings

Ingredients

- 4 catfish fillets
- 1 cup of yellow cornmeal
- 1 tbsp seasoned salt
- ¼ tsp pepper
- ¼ tsp garlic powder
- 1 cup of milk
- 3 tbsp vegetable oil
- 3 tbsp butter
- Parsley for garnish
- Lemon slices for garnish

Instructions

1. In a shallow bowl, combine the cornmeal, seasoned salt, pepper, and garlic powder.
2. Into a separate bowl, spill milk.

3. Over medium melt, heat the oil and butter in a large skillet.

4. Dip in the milk with a catfish fillet, and shake off some excess.

5. Transfer the milk-soaked fish to the mixture of cornmeal and spread carefully on both sides to cover.

6. For the remaining fillets, repeat.

7. Put the food in the hot skillet and cook on either side until golden brown (about 5-7 minutes per side) (about 5-7 minutes per side). With a fork, the fish will flake easily when it is done.

8. You will need to cook the fish in batches, depending on the size of your skillet.

9. The pan doesn't crowd! If applicable, for subsequent batches, feel free to rinse out the pan and use additional butter/oil.

10. On paper towels, drain fish.

11. Serve hot, if needed, garnished with chopped fresh parsley and a lemon wedge.

Nutrition

Calories: 222kcalFat: 15.8g

77.SPINACH DIP

Prep Time10 minutes

Cook Time20 minutes

Total Time30 minutes

Servings:10

INGREDIENTS

- 8 ounces cream softened cheese
- 1 cup ofcream sour
- 10 ounces leaves fresh spinach
- 1 tspgarlic minced
- 1/2salttsp
- 1/4peppertsp
- 1/2 cup ofgrated parmesan cheese
- 1 1/2 cups ofdivided usecheese shredded mozzarella
- 1 parsleychopped tbsp
- bread, crackers and vegetables for serving
- cooking spray

INSTRUCTIONS

1. Steam the spinach or saute it until wilted. Let it cool off then wring all the remaining moisture out. Chop the spinach coarsely.

2.with heat the oven to 375 degrees F. To line a shallow baking dish using cooking oil.

3. Place in a bowl the cream cheese, sour cream, cooked spinach, garlic, salt, pepper, parmesan and 3/4 cup mozzarella cheese. When well mixed, swirl.

4. Into the prepared bowl, scatter the spinach mixture. Cover with mozzarella cheese leftovers.

5. Bake for 20 minutes or until the cheese is melting and the dip is bubbly. Turn the oven to broil and cook for another 2-3 minutes or until the cheese is browning.

6. Sprinkle and eat with pizza, crackers and vegetables with minced parsley.

NUTRITION

Calories: 194kcal

Fat: 17g |

78.GRILLED GARLIC HERB ZUCCHINI

yield: 6 SERVINGSprep time: 15 MINUTEScook time: 10 MINUTEStotal time: 25 MINUTES

INGREDIENTS:

- 4 tbsp, divided olive oil
- 1/4 cup of minced shallot
- 2 cloves minced garlic
- 2 tbsp chopped fresh rosemary
- 2 tbsp chopped fresh parsley leaves
- Kosher salt and freshly ground black pepper, as need
- 2 medium zucchini, cut diagonally into 1/2-inch-thick slices
- 1 medium yellow squash, cut diagonally into 1/2-inch-thick slices
-

DIRECTIONS:

1. To medium high heat, preheat the barbecue.
2. In a small bowl, whisk together 3 tbsp olive oil, shallot, garlic, rosemary and parsley; season with salt and pepper, as need. Set back.
3. Brush zucchini and squash with remaining 1 tbsp olive oil; season with salt and pepper, as need.
4. Add to grill in a single layer, and cook until charred on both sides and only starting to soften, around 2 minutes per side.
5. Serve promptly, drizzled with olive oil mixture.

79.CINNAMON-ROASTED ALMONDS

Prep:15 mins

Cook:1 hr

Total:1 hr 15 mins

Servings:16

Ingredients

- 1 egg white
- 1 tsp cold water
- 4 cups of whole almonds
- ½ cup of white sugar
- ¼ tsp salt
- ½ tsp ground cinnamon

Directions

1. Preheat the boiler to 120 degrees C (250 degrees F) (120 degrees C). Lightly oil a 10x15 inch jellyroll bowl.

2. Lightly beat the white of the egg; add water and beat until frothy but not firm. Add the nuts, and blend until fully covered. Combine the sugar, cinnamon, and salt, and sprinkle over the nuts. Toss to cover, then sprinkle the prepared pan equally.

3. Bake in the preheated oven for 1 hour, stirring occasionally, until crispy. Allow to cool, then store in airtight containers of nuts.

Nutrition Facts

231 calories; fat 18g

80.CRISPY BAKED EGGPLANT
INGREDIENTS

- 2 pounds small to medium-size eggplant
- 2 large eggs
- 3/4 cup of finely grated Parmesan cheese
- 3/4 cup of plain panko breadcrumbs
- 1 tsp dried Italian Seasoning
- 1/2 tspevery kosher salt and freshly ground pepper
- Olive oil, for baking sheets
- Optional: marinara sauce for dipping

INSTRUCTIONS

1. To 375 degrees F. Preheat the oven. Brush the baking sheet vigorously with oil. Just set back. (Two sheets would need to be used.)

2. Whisk the eggs and 1 tablespoon of water in a small bowl. Combine the panko or Rice Chex crumbs, Parmesan, Italian seasoning, salt and pepper in another bowl (a pie plate works well).

3. Into thick rounds, cut the eggplants. (I like them to be between 1/2 and 3/4 inches thick, because before they get too fluffy, they have time to brown in the oven.) In the egg mixture, dip the eggplant slices, letting the excess run off. In the Parmesan sauce, dredge the dipped slices, pressing down softly to properly protect. To the baking tray, pass the coated slices.

4. Bake on the outside until golden brown, 17-20 minutes. (Use a spatula to peer underneath; if they're not yet crispy, give them a few more minutes and look again.) Turn the slices and proceed to bake on the other side until lightly browned but still slightly strong, about 10 minutes longer. Both ovens vary, so don't hesitate to change either direction for a few minutes. You tend to be golden brown on the first side, but care more of doneness and hue than make the second side equally brownish. (I simply gave the tops a fast broil when pressed for time, rather than flipping and cooking for the extra 10 minutes.)

5. Remove from the oven for dipping, and eat as is or with a side of marinara sauce.

NOTES

I recommend throwing the slices in a colander and tossing them with a half-tsp or so of salt if you would like to use this recipe with bigger eggplants. Allow for 20-30 minutes to drain the excess moisture, and then blot dry and proceed as instructed.

81.HEALTHY BAKED BROCCOLI TOTS

Prep Time: 15 minutesCook Time: 20 minutesTotal Time: 35 minutes Servings: 20 tots

Ingredients

- 2 cups of or 12 ounces uncooked or frozen broccoli
- 1 large egg
- 1/4 cup of diced yellow onion
- 1/3 cup of cheddar cheese
- 1/3 cup of panko breadcrumbs
- 1/3 cup ofitalian breadcrumbs
- 2 tbsp parsley
- 1/2 tsp salt
- 1/2 tsp pepper

Instructions

1. Preheat the boiler to 400°F. Grease and set aside a baking sheet with a thin layer of oil or line with parchment paper.

2. Blanch the broccoli for 1 minute in boiling water, then remove and shock to inhibit the cooking process with cold tap water. Drain thoroughly.

3. Finely cut the broccoli and combine it with the egg, onions, cheddar, breadcrumbs, and seasoning. Using an ice-cream scoop or your fingertips, scoop about 1.5 tbsp of mix, then gently press a strong ball between your hands and then create a tater-tot shape. After a handful, it helps to wash your hands

4. Tots to avoid them from sticking to your hand. Next place your lined baking sheet on top.

5. Bake 18-24 minutes until golden brown and crispy, turning halfway. With ketchup, sriracha, ranch dressing, or your favorite dipping sauce, remove it from the oven and eat it hot!

Nutrition

Calories: 26kcal |Fat: 1g

82.SKINNY JALAPEÑO POPPER DIP

Prep Time: 5 mins Cook Time: 10 mins Total Time: 15

INGREDIENTS

- 2 packages fat-free cream cheese, softened
- ½ C fat-free mayonnaise
- ½ tsp onion powder
- ½ tsp garlic powder
- ⅛ tsp salt
- ¼ C diced mild jalapeños, drained
- ½ C fat-free shredded sharp cheddar cheese

INSTRUCTIONS

1. Preheat oven to 375 degrees.
2. In a large bowl, blend together 8 oz melted cream cheese and ½ C fat-free mayonnaise until smooth.
3. Add 1/2 tsp of onion powder1/2 tsp of garlic powder 1/8 tsp of salt and 1/4 C of diced/drained jalapeños to the mixture..
4. Toss in ¼ C of the sliced strong cheddar cheese.
5. Pour mix into a shallow oven safe bowl, such as an 8x8 pan or baking dish.
6. Cover with remaining ¼ C of cheese.
7. Cook for 10-12 minutes, or until cheese is bubbly and melted.

8. Enjoy!

NOTES

- Serve hot, at room temperature, or freezing! Can be eaten with crackers, tortilla chips, or sliced vegetables.

Nutrition Facts

Total Fat 7.1g

83.SPICED NUTS

INGREDIENTS

- 1 tsp every cumin seeds, coriander seeds and fennel seeds
- 1 eggwhite
- 15 gm caster sugar
- 450 gm mixed nuts, such as raw cashews, natural almonds and unsalted peanuts
- 50 gm pumpkin seeds
- 2 tsp paprika
- 1 tsp dried chilli flakes
- Finely grated rind of 1 lemon

METHOD

1. Preheat the boiler to 150C. Pound all the spices in a mortar and pestle them until they are coarsely ground, then set aside.

2. In a wide bowl, whisk egg white until firm peaks form (1-2 minutes), add sugar gradually and whisk to combine. Stir in the remaining ingredients and 3 tsp of sea salt, spread on a baking sheet and roast, stirring periodically,

until golden (15-20 minutes) (15-20 minutes). Then break into pieces and serve. Set aside to cool. Spiced nuts will last for a week in an airtight jar.

84.VEGETABLE EGG ROLLS

Prep Time: 30 mins

Cook Time: 30 mins

Total Time: 1 hr

INGREDIENTS

- 1 Tbsp vegetable oil
- 1/2 tsp minced garlic
- 1 inch fresh ginger
- 4 oz. mushrooms
- 2 medium carrots
- 3 medium green onions
- 1 small head green cabbage
- 1/4 cup of soy sauce
- 1/2 Tbsp cornstarch
- 1 tsp sesame oil
- 1 pkg 20 ea egg roll wrappers
- as needed non-stick spray

INSTRUCTIONS

1. Cook the vegetables first. With a small holed cheese grater, peel the ginger and grind. Peel and grate a large holed cheese grater with the carrots. Mince the garlic (if

using fresh and not pre-minced garlic) (if using fresh rather than pre-minced). Dust and slice the mushrooms and green onions. Peel the cabbage's outer leaves, cut them into pieces, scrape the heart, and then slice them thinly into shreds.

2. Heat the vegetable oil over medium heat in a very large skillet or wok, and sauté the green onion, garlic and ginger until lightly softened (1-2 minutes) (1-2 minutes). Add the mushrooms and saute until the mushrooms are tender (about 5 minutes) (about 5 minutes). Add the carrot, add one more minute of saute, and add the cabbage. Continue to cook and stir until the volume of the cabbage has halved (increase the heat to medium-high if needed) (increase the heat to medium-high if necessary).

3. In the soy sauce, dissolve the cornstarch. To coat the vegetables, add them to the pan and mix. The heat would make it easier to thicken the mixture and create a glaze of soy sauce. Drizzle on top of sesame oil and stir in. Turn off the sun. Give the mixture a taste and, to your liking, change the soy sauce and sesame oil. To cool, move the mixture to a bowl.

4. Begin filling the egg rolls and rolling them. Place one wrapper on a clean surface at a time and place around 1/4 cup of the cabbage mixture just outside the middle, near one of the rectangle's corners. Roll up the corner and over the filling, fold either side in, and then roll up the rest of the way. Hold a little water bowl near by and use it as "glue" to secure the egg roll wrapper corners in place. (See below for step-by-step images)

5. To 425 degrees, preheat the oven. Create a baking sheet by covering it with foil. On the baking sheet, place

the egg rolls and coat them with non-stick oil. Roll them back and coat the other side (if you are opposed to non-stick spray, you should shave with vegetable oil). Bake for about 20 minutes or until golden brown and crispy in the fully preheated oven. If you have hot spots in your oven, transform the egg rolls halfway through cooking and rotate the baking sheet.

NUTRITION

Calories: 238.24kcalFat: 3.26g ·

85.STUFFED PORTOBELLO MUSHROOMS

Prep: 15 mins Cook: 25 mins Total: 40 mins Serves: 4

INGREDIENTS

- 4 large portobello mushrooms
- 1 tbsp olive oil
- 1/2chopped onion
- 4 cloves minced garlic
- 1/2 greenchopped bell pepper
- 2 cups ofchopped spinach
- 4 cocktailchopped tomatoes
- 1/4 cup of goat cheese crumbled
- 1/4 tsp salt or as need
- 1/4 tsp pepper or as need
- 1 tbsp hot sauce Frank's
- 1/2 cup of breadcrumbs
- 1/2 cup of mozzarella cheese

INSTRUCTIONS

1. Preheat the boiler to 400 degrees F.
2. Cautious removal of mushroom stems. Place the mushrooms stem side down into a baking pan. Bake for 10 to 15 minutes before the water spills out of them. Remove from the oven and using paper towels soak up excess water. Set back.
3. Do not throw away the stems from the mushrooms but cut them up to be added to the stuffing.
4. In a pan, melt the olive oil over low heat. Add the chopped onion and garlic and saute for a few minutes until the onion is translucent.
5. Add the green pepper and spinach to the skillet and simmer for a few of minutes. Add onions, goat cheese, salt, pepper, mushrooms roots, hot sauce and breadcrumbs. Stir and simmer for an extra few minutes.
6. Stuff the mushrooms with the mixture fairly. Cover with mozzarella sauce.
7. Bake for about 10 minutes or until the cheese melts.

RECIPE NOTES

- Please bear in mind that nutritional information is a rough approximation and can vary greatly depending on items used.

Nutrition Information:

Calories: 203kcaFat: 10g

86.YELLOW SQUASH FRITTERS

Prep Time:10 mins

Cook Time:20 mins

Total Time:30 mins

INGREDIENTS

- 1 lb. yellow squash, unpeeled
- ½ medium onion
- 1 large egg
- 1 tsp Diamond Crystal kosher salt
- ¼ tsp freshly ground black pepper
- 1 tsp garlic powder
- 2 tbsp unsalted butter for frying

INSTRUCTIONS

1. Using the shredding adapter, shred the squash in your food processor. Place it on clean towels and allow 10 minutes to drain. The squash can be grated by hand, too.

2. Cut the onion finely. Place it in a colander for 10 minutes to clean.

3. Over medium pressure, heat a large nonstick skillet for about 5 minutes.

4. Whisk the egg with cinnamon, black pepper and garlic powder in a medium bowl. Add the onion and the grated squash and blend to balance.

5. With half of the butter, brush the skillet. Spoon the mixture into the skillet, weighing half a cup in each fritter. Fry for 4-5

minutes without moving, before you can see that the bottoms are brown.

6. Flip to the other side cautiously and fry for 4-5 more minutes, before browning on both sides. With more sugar, wash the skillet and repeat with the remaining mixture of squash.

NOTES

Lacking starch, these are very delicate fritters. The more water you get out of the onion and squash, the more robust they'll be. In order to absorb the excess liquid, you can also try adding flour (if you do not like gluten) or coconut flour. Try coconut flour or 1/4 cup of all-purpose flour for 2 tbsp.

NUTRITION INFO

Low-carb (or keto) and gluten-free are the bulk of our dishes, but others are not. Before using it, please check that a recipe suits your needs. It is not assured that the recommended and related goods are gluten-free. The knowledge about diet is approximate and can include inconsistencies, so you can check it independently. It is measured using the calculator of the SparkPeople.com recipe and sugar alcohols are omitted from the carb count. Before using some of our recipes, read the disclaimers in our Terms of Use carefully..

Nutrition Facts

Fat7g

87.CREAMY SHRIMP CROQUETTES

Prep Time:15 mins

Cook Time:10 mins

Total Time:25 mins

Ingredients

- Creamy Shrimp Mixture
- 150g/5.3oz fresh medium size prawns/shrimps in shell
- 50g/1.8ozroughly chopped onion
- 300ml/10.1oz milk
- A couple of shakes of nutmeg powder
- 1 bay leaf
- ¼ tsp of salt
- Pepper
- 30g/1.1oz butter
- 40g/1.4oz flour
- Croquettes
- 2 tbsp flour
- 1beaten egg
- 1 cup of panko breadcrumbs
- Neutral oil for deep frying
- Serving
- Shredded cabbage
- 2 sprigs parsley

Instructions

1. Render the Creamy Shrimp Mixture.

2. Add to a saucepan the components of the Fluffy Shrimp Paste, minus butter and flour, and fire over medium high heat.

3. Turn the pan periodically as the surface of the milk begins to boil, so that the milk does not burn across the surface of the pan.

4. Turn the heat down to low and boil for a minute or before the prawns get red and rolled up, until the milk begins to simmer softly.

5. Withdraw from the heat and exit for an extra minute. Put the milk in a sieve and add it to the béchamel sauce.

6. Let the prawns cool down a bit, then peel the shells and cut the heads. Chop each prawn into 3-4 small bits.

7. Melt butter over low heat in a frying pan.

8. To mix properly, add rice. Cook for 3 minutes, stirring continually so that the color of the roux does not alter.

9. Add 1/3 of the reserved milk and mix well until lump free (note 2). (Remark 2).

10. In two batches, add surplus milk to the roux and mix together in the same direction.

11. To spread prawns evenly, add prawn bits and mix.

12. Transfer the mixture to a tray and shape it into a roughly 2.5cm/1" thick square.

13. To keep it from boiling up, cover the surface of the mixture with cling wrap. Let it cool off, so chill for a few hours in the refrigerator (note 3). (Remark 3).

Recipe Notes

- You would need 80g if you just have peeled prawns. The flavor of the prawns in the milk may not be as good.

- Using a whisk to clear lumps if needed.
- You should even cool it in the refrigerator. It would be OK to shape croquettes as long as the béchamel mixture becomes cool and firm.
- To deep fry three croquettes at a time, I used a shallow sauce pan. I placed another croquette on top of the one in the oil after lowering one croquette in the oil so that the croquette softly rolled into the oil.
- Creamy Shrimp Croquettes may be frozen either prior to deep frying or after deep frying. Keep frozen croquettes for about a month.

Nutrition

calories: 378kcal fat: 18g

88.EGGPLANT PARMIGIANA

Total: 2 hr 45 min

Prep: 35 min

Inactive: 1 hr

Cook: 1 hr 10 min

Yield: 4 and 6 servings

Ingredients

- Deselect All
- The Sauce:
- 1/4 cup of extra-virgin olive oil

- 3 medium yellow onions, peeled, halved, and cut into thin slices
- 6 cloves, peeled and grated garlic
- Kosher salt
- 1 tbsp crushed red pepper flakes
- 1 tbsp granulated sugar
- 3 cans San Marzano whole plum tomatoes
- The Eggplant:
- 2 medium eggplants, washed and cut into 1/2-inch thick rounds
- 1/2 cup of all-purpose flour
- Freshly ground black pepper
- 5 large eggs
- 3 tbsp whole milk
- 4 cups of Italian-style breadcrumbs
- 1 tbsp dried oregano
- 1 tbsp fresh thyme leave
- Vegetable oil, for frying, as needed, about 1 1/2 to 2 cups of
- 1 1/2 pounds mozzarella cheese, cut into thin slices
- 1/2 cup of grated Parmesan
- 1 pound , grated provolone cheese
- 2 handfuls fresh basil, leaves only, torn

Directions

1. Render the Creamy Shrimp Mixture

2. Add to a saucepan the components of the Fluffy Shrimp Paste, minus butter and flour, and fire over medium high heat.

3. Turn the pan periodically if the milk surface is bubbling, so that the milk does not burn over the surface of the pan.

4. Turn the heat down to low and boil for a minute or before the prawns get red and rolled up, until the milk begins to simmer gently.

5. Withdraw from the heat and exit for an extra minute. Place the milk in a sieve and reserve it for the béchamel sauce.

6. Let the prawns cool down a little, then scrape the shells and cut the heads. Chop one prawn into 3-4 little sections.

7. Melt butter in a frying pan over low heat.

8. To blend well add rice. Cook for 3 minutes, stirring continuously so that there is no color difference in the roux.

9. Add 1/3 of the reserved milk and blend well before lump clear, to be added (note 2). (Remark 2). (Remark 2).

10. In two batches, add the remaining milk to the roux and blend together in the same direction.

11. To disperse prawns uniformly, add prawn bits and merge.

Transfer the mixture to a tray and shape it into a roughly 2.5cm/1" thick square

12. In order to prevent it from heating up, cover the surface of the blend with cling wrap. Let it cool first, so relax for a few hours in the refrigerator (note 3). (Remark 3). (Remark 3).

Recipe Notes

- You would like 80g if you just had peeled prawns. The flavor of prawns in milk isn't going to be as sweet.
- Using a whisk to clear lumps if needed.

- You should even cool it in the refrigerator. It would be OK to shape croquettes as long as the béchamel mixture becomes cool and stable.
- To deep fry three croquettes at a time, I used a shallow sauce pan. I put another croquette on top of the one in the oil after lowering one croquette in the oil so that the croquette softly rolled into the oil.
- Creamy Shrimp Croquettes may be frozen either prior to deep frying or after deep frying. Hold frozen croquettes for about a month

89.EASY CHICKEN CHIMICHANGAS

Prep Time15 minutes

Cook Time6 minutes

Total Time21 minutes

Servings8

Ingredients

- cooking oil
- 1 rotisserie chicken
- 8 10" tortillas
- 15 ounces can black beans
- 1 1/2 cups of rice cooked
- 1 1/2 cups of shredded colby jack cheese
- 1/2 cup of homemade salsa
- 1 tbsp chili powder
- 2 tsp cumin
- 1 tsp salt

Instruction

1. Preheat a frying pan over medium-high heat with around 1/2" cooking oil.

2. Laid out the tortillas on a flat surface. Divide the beans and rice equally between them.

3. Blend the shredded chicken, sauce, and spices in a small bowl, and add them evenly to the tortillas.

4. Top each tortilla with grilled cheese, and roll up as you go, folding the sides.

5. In the hot oil, add the chimichangas, frying 2-3 at a time. Turn from 2-3 minutes after the bottom has browned.

6. Cook until completely browned, then drain on paper towels.

7. Instantly serve.

Notes

- Cover with chopped broccoli, onions, avocado, and sour cream to eat.
- The calories shown are based on 8 chimichangas, with 1 serving being 1 chimichanga, based on the recipe. Since various ingredient labels have different nutritional records, the calories displayed are only an estimation of calories..

Nutrition

Calories: 754kcalFat: 28g

90.BUFFALO CAULIFLOWER

Prep:15 mins

Cook:30 mins

Additional:10 mins

Total:55 mins

Servings:4

Ingredients

- olive oil cooking spray
- ¾ cup of gluten-free baking flour
- 1 cup of water
- ½ tsp garlic powder, or as need
- salt and ground black pepper as need
- 2 heads cauliflower, cut into bite-size pieces
- 2 tbsp butter
- ½ cup of hot pepper sauce
- 1 tsp honey

DirectionsInstructions

1. Preheat the boiler to 230 degrees C (450 degrees F) (230 degrees C). Oil the baking sheet lightly with sauce to cook.

2. Use a whisk to mix flourwater, garlic powdersalt and pepper in a bowl until the batter is smooth and slightly runny. Add the flour to the cauliflower and blend until the cauliflower is coated; spread on the baking sheet.

3. Bake in the preheated oven for 20 to 25 minutes until well browned.

4. In a saucepan, melt butter with over low heat. Remove the sauce from the fire and stir the butter with the sweet pepper sauce and honey until smooth. Brush the mixture of hot sauce over each slice of cauliflower and repeat brushing until all the mixture of hot sauce is used.

5. Bake in the oven for 10 minutes until the cauliflower has browned. Remove the baking sheet from the oven and give 10 to 15 minutes for the cauliflower to cool.

Cook's Note:

- Gluten-free flour uses less liquid than wheat flour. You will have to change the liquid depending on the flour you are using.
- All-purpose flour can be used in place of gluten-free if desired.

Nutrition Facts

218 calories fat 7.1g;

91.AIR FRYER STEAK BITES & MUSHROOMS

Prep Time10 mins

Cook Time18 mins

Total Time28 mins

INGREDIENTS

- 1 lb. steaks cut into 1/2" cubes
- 8 oz. mushrooms
- 2 Tbspmelted Butter
- 1 tsp Worcestershire sauce
- 1/2 tsp garlic powder optional
- flakey salt as need
- fresh cracked black pepper as need
- Minced parsley garnish
- Melted butter optional for finishing
- Chili Flakesfor finishing optional

INSTRUCTIONS

1. Rinse the steak cubes and thoroughly pat them dry. Combine the cubes and mushrooms with the beef. Coat with melted butter and season with Worcestershire sauce garlic powder optional, and salt and pepper seasoning.

2. For 4 minutes preheat the Air Fryer at 400°F.

3. In the air fryer basket scatter the steak and the mushrooms in an even layer. Fry for 10-18 minutes at 400 ° F shake and flip and fry the steak and mushrooms twice during the frying process (time depends on the ideal doneness steak thickness air

fryer size) (time depends on your preferred donenessthickness of the steak size of air fryer).

4. Check the steak to see how good it is cooked and done. Add an extra 2-5 minutes of cooking time if you want the steak grilled better.

5. Garnish with parsley and drizzle with optional chili flakes and/or optional melted butter. If needed season with additional salt & pepper. Wet to serve.

NOTES

- Recipes in 3-4 qt air fryers have been measured. The recipe can cook faster if you use a larger air fryer so adjust the cooking time.
- The first batch would take longer to cook if it was prepared in multiple batches and not pre-heated before the first batch.
- It is preferable to preheat the Air Fryer. Add more time to the cooking if you do not preheat.
- Remember to set a shake/flip/toss timer for the food as directed in the recipe.
- Course: Main Cooking Course: Air Fryer

NUTRITION

Calories: 29gl

Fat:401kca

92.CHICKEN TIKKA KEBAB

Prep Time: 35 mins

Cook Time: 15 mins

Total Time: 50 mins

Servings: 4

INGREDIENTS

- 1 lb Chicken thighs boneless skinless, cut into 1.5-2 inch cubes
- 1 tbsp Oil
- ½ cup of Red Onion cut into 2 inch cubes, layers separated
- ½ cup of Green Bell Pepper cut into 2 inch cubes
- ½ cup of Red Bell Pepper cut into 2 inch cubes
- Lime wedges to garnish
- Onion rounds to garnish
- For marinade
- ½ cup of Yogurt greek
- ¾ tbspgrated Ginger
- ¾ tbspminced Garlic
- tbsp Lime juice
- tsp Kashmiri red chili powder mild, adjust as need
- ½ tsp Ground Turmeric
- tsp Garam Masala
- 1 tsp Coriander powder
- ½ tbsp Dried Fenugreek leaves
- tsp Salt adjust as need

INSTRUCTIONS

1. Combine all ingredients for the marinade in a bowl and blend well. Add chicken and coat on either hand with the marinade. Let it rest for anything from 30 minutes and 8 hours in the refrigerator.
2. When ready to serve, add the oil, onions, green and red bell pepper to the marinade. Mix well.
3. Thread the marinated chicken, peppers and onions in the skewers altenating between every.

NOTES

- Tips to Make the Perfect Chicken Tikka
- Marinate: Marinate for at least 30 minutes, but longer is best for more tender Chicken Tikka.
- Cook: For better results cook the meat only until cooked. This will result in soft, juicy & tender chicken kebabs. Over cooked meat can result in chewy kebabs.
- Meal Prep: Produce a batch of this marinated chicken and freeze for later use or meal prep for the week.
- Skewers: I used wooden skewers which I soaked in water for 30 minutes and cut them in a smaller size so they would fit in the air fryer or in the crisplid basket. You can use bamboo skewers too.
- Make Chicken Tikka Bites: Avoid the skewers and place the marinated chicken and veggies directly in the air fryer basket to make chicken tikka bites.

NUTRITION

Calories: 337kcal

Fat: 24g

93. CRISPY AIR FRIED TOFU

Prep: 30 minutes Cook: 15 minutes Total: 45 minutes

Ingredients

- 1 16-oz block extra-firm tofu 453 g
- 2 Tbsp soy sauce 30 mL
- 1 Tbsp toastedoil 15 mL sesame
- 1 Tbsp15 mL olive oil
- 1 clove minced garlic

Instructions

1. Press: Press tofu for at least 15 minutes, using either an or by placing a heavy pan on top of it, letting the moisture drain. When done, cut tofu into bite-sized blocks and transfer to a bowl.
2. Flavor: Mix the remaining ingredients in a shallow bowl. Drizzle over tofu and throw to cover. Let the tofu marinate for 15 more minutes.
3. AirFry: Preheat the air fryer to 375 degrees F (190 C) (190 C). Add tofu blocks to your air fryer basket in a single sheet. Cook for 10 to 15 minutes, shaking the pan occasionally to facilitate even cooking.

Nutrition Information

Calories: 165kcal Fat: 1.9g

94.BUTTERED COD FISH RECIPE

Prep Time: 5 minutesCook Time: 5 minutesTotal Time: 10 minutes

Servings: 4 servings

INGREDIENTS

- cod-

- 1 1/2 lbs cod fillets
- 6 Tbspsliced unsalted butter,
- seasoning-
- ¼ tsp garlic powder
- ½ tsp salt
- ¼ tsp ground black pepper
- ¾ tsp ground paprika
- 1 tsp fresh herbs
- few lemon slices, drizzle for serving
- US Customary – Metric

INSTRUCTIONS

1. Combine the ingredients for the seasoning in a shallow bowl.
2. Cut cod into smaller bits, if desired. Season both sides of the cod with the seasoning.
3. Heat 2 Tbsp butter in a large skillet with over medium-high heat. Add cod to the skillet as the butter melts. Cook 2 minutes.

4. Turn the heat down to medium. Gently flip the cod. Cover with remaining butter and cook for 3-4 minutes.
5. Butter will absolutely melt and the fish will cook. (Don't overcook the cod, it will get mushy and totally fall apart.)
6. Drizzle cod with fresh lemon juice and spices. Serve instantly.
7. Enjoy, mates.

NUTRITION

Calories: 294kcaFat: 18g

95.15 MINUTE THAI BASIL CHICKEN

Prep Time: 6 mins Cook Time: 9 mins Total Time: 15 minutes

INGREDIENTS

- 2 tbsp vegetable oil
- 3 tbsp oyster sauce
- 2 tbsp soy sauce
- 2 tbsp fish sauce
- 3 tbsp sugar
- 1 red bellchopped pepper,
- 8 ounces green beans
- 1 1/2 pounds boneless,, coarsely choppe skinless chicken thighs
- 4 sliced shallots
- 4 cloves minced garlic
- 4 minced Thai chilies, or as need
- 1 cup of very thinly sliced fresh Thai basil leaves
- Jasmine rice, to serve

INSTRUCTIONS

1. Heat the oil in a wok or heavy, high-walled skillet with over high heat. If the wok is heating up, whisk together the oyster sauce, soy sauce, fish sauce, and sugar until well-combined. Set back.
2. Add the bell pepper and green beans to the hot wok. Stir-fry for one minute. Add in the chicken and stir-fry, breaking apart as you go, before starting to brown, about 2 minutes.
3. Stir in the shallots, ginger, and Thai chilies. Cook for 1 more minute, before fragrant. Then, add in the cooked sauce. Continue to cook until the sauce starts to glaze onto the beef, around 1-2 more minutes.
4. Stir in the Thai basil leaves and simmer until the chicken is fully cooked through, the basil is wilted, and the liquid has almost evaporated. Serve warm with rice.

96.ONE PAN MEATBALL CASSEROLE

prep Time: 10 minutesCook Time: 50 minutesTotal Time: 1 hourServings:8

Ingredients

- 16 oz. package uncooked ziti pasta
- 24 ounces marinara sauce
- 1 cup of milk
- 2 cups of water
- 1/2 tsp garlic powder
- 1/2 tsp onion powder
- 1 tsp oregano
- 1 tsp salt

- Meatballs , fully cooked, thawed
- 2 cups of shredded mozzarella
- Optional: Parmesan cheese and fresh chopped herbs

Instructions

1. Preheat oven to 425 degrees F.
2. In a 9x13 inch baking dish stir together uncooked spaghetti, marinara sauce, water, milk, spices and meatballs.
3. Cover securely with aluminium foil and bake for 40 minutes.
4. Uncover; stir. Test the pasta for doneness. We want it to be al dente (firm, yet almost perfectly cooked) (firm, but almost perfectly cooked). If its still too hard cover the dish and return to the oven for a few minutes.
5. 5. Spread mozzarella over the top and bake for another 5-10 minutes or until uncovered. cheese is melted and bubbly.
6. Allow to cool for at least 15 minutes before eating, to allow the sauce to thicken up.

Notes

- Want to produce a smaller batch? Cut the recipe in half and bake in an 8" or equivalent size bowl.
- Make Ahead: This recipe may be assembled entirely the night before, but I wouldn't do it any earlier than that or the noodles can have a mushy feel after baking.
- Freezing Instructions: Cook the recipe up to baking. Cover with a double coat of aluminium foil and ice for up to 3 months. Thaw in the freezer before baking, or to bake from froze, baked covered for 1 hour and 30 minutes, and uncovered for 15-20 minutes longer.

- Slow Cooker: Prepare as directed, just leave out the milk and add an extra 24 oz container of marinara sauce. Be sure the ziti noodles are filled with sauce. Cook for 2 - 2 1/2 hours on HIGH, or for 3 1/3 hours on LOW-4 hours or until pasta is tender. During the last few minutes of preparation, sprinkle mozzarella cheese on top and return the lid to allow the cheese to melt. Optional-place under broiler for a few minutes to toast the cheesy top.

Nutrition

Calories: 335kca Fat: 8g

97.TABASCO GRILLED SHRIMP

Prep Time 20 MINUTESCook Time 10 MINUTESServings 2
SERVINGS

INGREDIENTS

- 1 lb largepeeled, deveined shrimp
- 2 tbsp olive oil
- 1 tsp Tabasco sauce
- 1 tbsp fresh thyme
- 1/2 tsp kosher salt
- 1/2 tsp cracked black pepper

INSTRUCTIONS

1. Toss all ingredients together and allow to marinate at room temperature for around 15 minutes.
2. Loop the shrimp into barbecue skewers.

3. Grill over medium-high heat for around 3 minutes per
   hand. Serve and enjoy.

NUTRITION

Calories: 355kcaFat: 17g

98.LEMON PEPPER COD

Prep:5 mins

Cook:10 mins

Total:15 mins

Servings:4

Ingredients

- 3 tbsp vegetable oil
- 1 ½ pounds fillets cod
- 1 lemon juiced
- ground blackas need pepper

Directions

1. In a broad skillet, heat oil over medium high heat until
   hot. Add the fillets then squeeze over the tops with 1/2 of
   the lemon juice. Sprinkle with pepper if need. Cook for 4
   minutes and transform. Squeeze with the remaining
   lemon's juice and sprinkle with pepper if need. Continue
   to cook until fillets flake quickly with a for
2. Towards Directions Checklist guidelines
3. In a broad skillet, heat oil over medium high heat until hot
   .Add the fillets then squeeze over the tops with 1/2 of the
   lemon juice. Sprinkle with pepper if need. Cook for 4

minutes and transform. Squeeze with the remaining lemon's juice and sprinkle with pepper if need. Continue to cook until fillets flake quickly with a for.

Nutrition Facts

236 calories;

fat 11.5g;

99.ZESTY RANCH AIR FRYER FISH FILLETS

Prep Time:5 minutes

Cook Time:12 minutes

Total Time:17 minutes

Ingredients

- 3/4 cup of bread crumbs or Panko or crushed cornflakes
- 1 30g packet dry ranch-style dressing mix
- 2 1/2 tbsp vegetable oil
- 2 beaten eggs
- 4 tilapia salmon or other fish fillets
- lemon wedges to garnish

Instructions

1. 1. Preheat the 180 degree air fryer to C.
2. Blend together the panko/breadcrumbs and the combination of ranch dressing.Add the oil and keep stirring until the mixture becomes crumbly and loose.
3. Dip the fish fillets into the egg, letting the excess run off.
4. Dip the fish fillets into the crumb paste, making sure to cover them uniformly and thoroughly.
5. Place into your air fryer carefully.

6. Depending on the thickness of the fillets, 6. Cook for 12-13 minutes.
7. Remove and serve. Squeeze the lemon wedges over the fish if needed.

Nutrition Information

Calories: 315kcaFat: 14g

100.PAN-SEARED COD IN WHITE WINE TOMATO BASIL SAUCE

prep 15 minscook 25 minstotal 40 mins

Ingredients

- For the White Wine Tomato Basil Sauce:
- 2 tbsp olive oil
- 1/4 tsp crushed red pepper flakes
- 3 large, finely minced cloves garlic
- 1 pint cherry tomatoes, sliced in half
- 1/4 cup of dry white wine
- 1/2 cup of, finely chopped fresh basil
- 2 tbsp fresh lemon juice
- 1/2 tsp fresh lemon zest
- 1/2 tsp salt
- 1 tsp granulated sugar
- 1/4 tsp fresh ground black pepper
- For the Cod
- 2 tbsp olive oil
- 1 and 1/2 pounds fresh cod, cut into 4 fillets
- Salt and pepper

Instructions

1. For the White Wine Basil Sauce of Tomatoes:

2. Heat oil with over a medium heat in a large saute pan. Add the flakes of crushed red pepper and garlic and saute for 1 minute or until the garlic is fragrant. Add the cherry tomatoes and cook for 9 to 12 minutes, stirring occasionally, until soft and blistering, while still maintaining their form. Add the white wine, stir, and allow the mixture to boil lovingly. Add the basil, lemon juice, lemon zest, salt, sugar and pepper to the mixture and boil for about 2 minutes. In a bowl, transfer the sauce and set it aside until necessary.

3. Concerning the Cod:

4. Heat oil with over a medium heat in a large saute pan. Pat the cod with paper towels to dry up. Then season the cod with salt and pepper on both sides.

5. Place the cod in the oil and cook for about 3 minutes until it is golden brown. Flip the cod over cautiously and continue to cook for another 3 to 4 minutes, OR until it is cooked through.

6. Pour over the cod the white wine tomato basil sauce, allow the sauce to warm for a minute, then remove from the heat and serve immediately.

Notes

- The cooking process of this recipe has been changed somewhat. There is also the same recipe and taste!

101.BAKED SEA BASS WITH FENNEL

Prep:15 mins

Cook:30 mins

Serves 2

Ingredients

- 2 smallscaled and gutted sea bass ,
- 1 fennelslicedbulb ,
- 1sliced lemon
- handful basil leaves , roughly torn
- small handful black olives
- 1 tbsp olive oil

Method

1. 200C/180C fan/gas heating appliance 6. Rinse the fish and rinse it out. Season all over, and then cram some fennel slices, lemon and basil into the cavity. In a roasting pan, sprinkle the olives and any remaining fennel, basil and lemon together.
2. Place the bass in the sea on top. Drizzle with the oil on any fish and bake for about 30 minutes or until cooked through and browned.

102.GARLIC LEMON SHRIMP

Ingredients

- for 2 servings

- 3 tbsp butter
- 1 lb shrimp deveined with tails removed
- 1 tsp salt
- ½ tsp pepper
- 3 cloves minced garlic
- ½ tsp red chili flakes
- 1 tbsp chopped fresh parsley,
- 3 tbsp lemon juice

Preparation

1. Melt butter over medium heat in a casserole bowl.
2. Spread the shrimp in a single layer around the plate, sprinkle the salt and pepper on top, then cook until the butter starts to turn a dark brown colour. Flip the shrimp, add the flakes of garlic and chili, then simmer for 15-30 seconds or so.
3. Add the parsley and lemon juice to the sauce, reduce the amount of lemon juice and then remove from the heat.
4. Serving and loving it!